Praise for
TRANSFORMING TODDLERHOOD

"True transformation happens when we stop seeing toddler behaviors as problems to fix and start seeing them as opportunities to grow. Devon provides the perfect blend of conscious parenting wisdom and real-world tools, giving parents everything they need to stay connected and calm in their most challenging moments."

—**Dr. Shefali Tsabary,** *New York Times* bestselling author of *The Conscious Parent* and *The Awakened Family*

"Stymied by a toddler? Here's a comprehensive resource for parents who are wondering what's normal, what's not, and what to do about it."

—**Joanna Faber and Julie King,** coauthors of *How to Talk So LITTLE Kids Will Listen: A Survival Guide to Life with Children Ages 2–7*

"*Transforming Toddlerhood* is a deeply insightful and practical almanac for anyone determined to create a secure experience for their child through some of life's messiest and most delightful years."

—**Eli Harwood,** MA, LPC, bestselling author of *Raising Securely Attached Kids*

"More than anything, *Transforming Toddlerhood* is a toolkit. Parents can come back to it again and again to help them navigate the power struggles, big emotions, and growing independence that come with this important stage of development."

—**Jessica Rolph,** cofounder and CEO of Lovevery

"I call the twos the 'teachable twos,' and Devon thinks the same. In *Transforming Toddlerhood*, she gives you practical scripts and tools to stay calm, hold space, and truly understand what's underneath the meltdown. As a mom of twins who's learned that emotional regulation starts with your own emotional regulation and presence, I found this book to be a game changer."

—**Hilary Swank,** actress, storyteller, mom of twins

"This is the guide I *wish* I'd had when my daughter was a toddler! Devon Kuntzman is the Toddler Whisperer, and she shares all her secrets in this very clear and digestible guide. Devon's approach is exactly the compassionate and firm perspective that toddler parents need to create positive, life-long relationships. With easy-to-follow bite-sized lessons, *Transforming Toddlerhood* will help the most sleep-deprived toddler parent. From a Mindful Parenting perspective, I heartily endorse *Transforming Toddlerhood!*"

—**Hunter Clarke-Fields,** bestselling author of *Raising Good Humans* and host of the *Mindful Mama Podcast*

"It's a great book to refer to when you feel stuck with your toddler—calm, respectful, and very aligned with Montessori values."

—**Simone Davies,** author of *The Montessori Toddler*

"A straightforward and empowering guide for parents, this book offers practical tools to regulate your own emotions while helping your toddler learn to do the same. Compassionate in tone, while grounded in research, it's a gift to every overwhelmed parent and caregiver. A must-read for anyone who wants to raise emotionally healthy kids while nurturing their own well-being."

—**Christopher Willard,** PhD, Harvard Medical School, author of *Growing Up Mindful, Alphabreaths,* and *Feelings are Like Farts*

"Raising resilient, thriving kids starts with connection—not control. As a holistic pediatrician, I see how overwhelmed parents can feel navigating tantrums, power struggles, sensory overload, and emotional meltdowns. In *Transforming Toddlerhood*, Devon Kuntzman offers a compassionate, science-backed road map that helps parents navigate toddlerhood with clarity, connection, and confidence. A must-read for every parent who wants to support their child's emotional well-being from the start."

—**Dr. Elisa Song,** MD, integrative pediatrician and bestselling author of *Healthy Kids, Happy Kids*

"Rooted in solid brain science and deep respect for both kids and their caregivers, *Transforming Toddlerhood* makes big concepts like emotional regulation feel clear and offers practical strategies you can start using today. Devon shows you that toddlerhood isn't just a difficult phase to survive—she explains why toddlers do what they do and how to respond in ways that actually help (without making you feel like you've been doing it all wrong). This book will help you see your child's behavior with more understanding, respond with more calm and confidence, and even enjoy this wild ride a little more."

—**Lane Rebelo,** LCSW, best-selling author of *Baby Sign Language Made Easy*

"Toddlers aren't tiny tyrants—they're just little humans with big feelings and undeveloped brains. In *Transforming Toddlerhood*, Devon Kuntzman doesn't sugarcoat the chaos but shows you how to meet it with connection, clarity, and calm. This book respects parents' instincts, offers real tools that work, and reminds you that discipline isn't about control—it's about teaching. A refreshingly grounded guide for anyone in the thick of toddlerhood."

—**Jamie Glowacki,** author of *Oh Crap! I Have a Toddler* and *Oh Crap! Potty Training*

"*Transforming Toddlerhood* illuminates what so much parenting advice misses: toddlers aren't misbehaving—they're communicating! With clarity and warmth, Devon Kuntzman helps parents understand the 'why' behind the behavior so they can respond with empathy, set respectful limits, and build the emotional safety toddlers need to thrive. Rooted in child development and the principles of peaceful parenting, this book gives parents practical tools, emotional insight, and a deep understanding of what young children truly need to grow up emotionally healthy and resilient."

—**Dr. Laura Markham,** clinical psychologist and author of *Peaceful Parent, Happy Kids*

"This book beautifully bridges the science of early childhood with the heart of parenting. Devon offers thoughtful reflections and guidance that can help parents feel more grounded and supported through the ups and downs of toddlerhood."

—**Susan Stiffelman,** MFT, author of *Parenting Without Power Struggles*

TRANSFORMING TODDLERHOOD

TRANSFORMING TODDLERHOOD

How to Handle Tantrums, End Power Struggles, and Raise Resilient Kids—
Without Losing Your Mind

DEVON KUNTZMAN

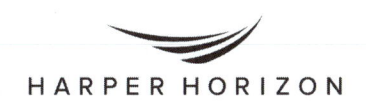

HARPER HORIZON

Transforming Toddlerhood

Copyright © 2025 by Devon Kuntzman

All rights reserved. No portion of this book may be reproduced, stored in a retrieval system, or transmitted in any form or by any means—electronic, mechanical, photocopy, recording, scanning, or other—except for brief quotations in critical reviews or articles, without the prior written permission of the publisher.

Published by Harper Horizon, an imprint of HarperCollins Focus LLC, 501 Nelson Place, Nashville, TN 37214, USA.

Any internet addresses, phone numbers, or company or product information printed in this book are offered as a resource and are not intended in any way to be or to imply an endorsement by Harper Horizon, nor does Harper Horizon vouch for the existence, content, or services of these sites, phone numbers, companies, or products beyond the life of this book.

The information contained in this book is for general informational and educational purposes only and is not intended as a substitute for professional advice, diagnosis, or treatment. Always consult with qualified professionals regarding any concerns or decisions that may affect your child's health, well-being, or development. The author and publisher disclaim any liability for any adverse effects resulting directly or indirectly from the application of any information presented in this book.

Names and identifying characteristics of some individuals have been changed to preserve their privacy.

ISBN 978-1-4002-5296-1 (ePub)
ISBN 978-1-4002-5295-4 (HC)

Without limiting the exclusive rights of any author, contributor, or the publisher of this publication, any unauthorized use of this publication to train generative artificial intelligence (AI) technologies is expressly prohibited. HarperCollins also exercise their rights under Article 4(3) of the Digital Single Market Directive 2019/790 and expressly reserve this publication from the text and data mining exception.

HarperCollins Publishers, Macken House, 39/40 Mayor Street Upper, Dublin 1, D01 C9W8, Ireland (https://www.harpercollins.com)

Library of Congress Control Number: 2025938658

Art director: Belinda Bass
Cover design: Mary Catherine Starr
Interior design: Kait Lamphere

Printed in Canada

25 26 27 28 29   TC   5 4 3 2 1

For my son—my tiniest teacher, full-time
mischief-maker, and spark of everyday magic.

And for my husband—my steadfast teammate,
wrangler of wild mornings, and the one who
shows up, even when the cereal hits the fan.

This is for the laughter, the love, and the life we've built.
Together, you are my greatest adventure.

CONTENTS

Foreword by Tina Payne Bryson, PhD xv

Introduction: The Truth About Toddlerhood

1. Welcome to Transforming Toddlerhood 3
2. What Is a Toddler and How Do You Know You Have One? 9
3. Toddlers Aren't Terrible 15
4. How to Use This Book 21

Part 1: The Toddler Parent

5. Establishing Positive, Effective, Developmentally
   Appropriate Parenting 29
6. Understanding Your Parenting Role 35
7. Doing the Internal Work of Parenting 43
8. Becoming a Safe Parent 48
9. Cultivating Patience and Preventing Burnout 55
10. Parenting Together 63

Part 2: The Toddler Explained

11. Understanding the Toddler Brain 73
12. Getting to Know Your Toddler's Sensory System 80
13. Setting Realistic Expectations 87
14. Decoding Toddler Behavior 94

CONTENTS

15. Redefining Discipline. 101
16. Building Connection 115
17. Setting Limits. 123
18. Teaching Skills 132

Part 3: The Emotional Toddler

19. Calming an Upset Toddler 141
20. Transforming Tantrums 156
21. Understanding Crying 169
22. Decoding Screaming, Yelling, and Demands 176
23. Responding to Whining. 184
24. Addressing Hurtful Words 191
25. Coping with Parental Preference 198
26. Navigating Screen Time Confidently. 205
27. Disarming Power Struggles 218
28. Handling Transitions 226
29. Building Your Child's Confidence 231

Part 4: The Physical Toddler

30. Cultivating Consent and Body-Safety Skills. 241
31. Stopping Aggressive Behavior 250
32. Overcoming Sleep Challenges 259
33. Brushing and Caring for Teeth .270
34. Teaching Toilet-Learning Skills .278
35. Ending Mealtime Chaos 293
36. Balancing Safety and Exploration 304
37. Playing Independently 311

Part 5: The Social Toddler

38. Modeling Manners 325
39. Addressing Lying 334
40. Easing Separation Anxiety 339

CONTENTS

41. Supporting a Slow-to-Warm-Up (Shy) Child..............346
42. Managing Sibling Conflict................................353
43. Cultivating Sharing Skills 360
44. Raising a Helper..369
45. Welcoming a New Baby 376

Conclusion: There Is No Such Thing as Failure................385

Acknowledgments..389
Notes 391
Index 401
About the Author...409

FOREWORD

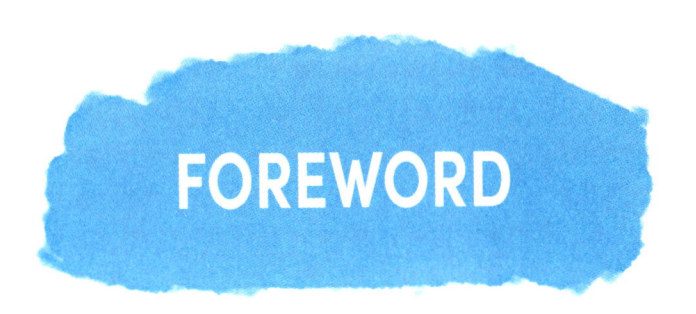

Toddlerhood can humble even the most well-read, well-prepared parent (or child development expert!). It's a season full of contradictions: exhilarating and exhausting, heart-melting and hair-pulling, joyful and deeply overwhelming—sometimes all in the same five minutes.

In my nearly three decades as a pediatric psychotherapist, educator, parenting author, and mother to three boys (now young adults), I've experienced and witnessed this parental roller coaster countless times. I've sat with exhausted parents who felt like failures because their two-year-old had yet another public meltdown. I've watched families become trapped in cycles of power struggles that left everyone feeling defeated. And I've listened as parents shared the guilt they felt because they weren't enjoying parenting their three- or four-year-old. Yet, when I asked them to tell me something funny or cute their child had done recently, their faces would light up. Every parent's story is unique and complex, and there's never a one-size-fits-all approach. But one thing so many families have in common is that these challenges often stem from a fundamental misunderstanding of what's really happening in their toddler's developing brain.

This mismatch between our expectations and what toddlers are experiencing developmentally is one reason so many families struggle during these years. Parents feel like they're constantly battling their child, and toddlers feel misunderstood, frustrated, and overwhelmed. The cultural narrative that toddlerhood is "terrible" only reinforces the idea that these years are something to endure, rather than a remarkable period of growth and discovery to embrace.

Through my work in interpersonal neurobiology—studying how the brain changes through relational experiences—and years of research on brain development, attachment, and emotional regulation, I know this truth intimately: Toddlerhood is a pivotal time when a child's brain is rapidly wiring for connection, regulation, empathy, resilience, and thousands of other capacities. The behaviors that drive you to the edge of sanity—the defiance, the meltdowns, the seemingly irrational reactions and demands—are actually signs of healthy development.

The kind of blossoming happening in your little one's brain during these years is one of the most sophisticated processes in the known universe. What many parents don't realize, though, is that development isn't linear—it involves regressions alongside progressions. And it's not synchronous either. When children experience a burst of growth in one domain, it doesn't mean all domains are growing at the same pace. Cognitive development, for example, doesn't always align with motor, emotional, or social development. Big ideas? Yes. Big emotional agility? Not yet. One of my own three-year-olds sobbed for a good ten minutes because he couldn't "walk up the wall like Spider-Man."

Typically, between eighteen months and three years, children experience a profound growth spurt in the left hemisphere of the brain: Language comes online, they begin to understand cause and effect, and they are driven to know "why." But here's the challenge: Just because they can say, "I want the red plate," doesn't mean they have the emotional-regulation skills to handle it when the red plate is in the dishwasher. Essentially, toddlers are walking around with big feelings and very little ability to manage them. It's like having the gas pedal pressed down without quite knowing how to use the brakes. No wonder the red plate "crisis" feels like the end of the world to them.

What makes *Transforming Toddlerhood* so helpful is not just its deep grounding in child development, attachment science, and neuroscience, but Devon's gift for translation. Three messages I return to repeatedly in my books—that behavior is communication; that regulation skills come primarily from brain development and repeated co-regulation experiences with a safe, predictable, positive grown-up; and that parents need to be both in charge and emotionally responsive—are not only honored in these pages but applied to everyday moments with toddlers, even down to toothbrushing and potty learning.

While many books gloss over these early years or treat toddlers as mini versions of older children, Devon has created an incredibly comprehensive guide specifically for the unique challenges and opportunities of this phase (ages one through five). She honors both the developmental needs of children *and* parents' desire for cooperation and connection. With bite-size chapters, real-world scripts, and "toddler tips," her practical approach makes it possible for overwhelmed parents (are those two words redundant?) to find exactly what they need, exactly when they need it most. This book doesn't just tell you what to do; it shows you how to show up with presence, boundaries, and empathy—even when your child is throwing a shoe at your face with shockingly athletic precision.

The pages ahead will feel like sitting down with a trusted guide who sees the chaos, the tears, the tantrums—and the sacredness hidden within them. And what a relief: Devon doesn't flinch from the hard stuff. She names the moments every toddler parent knows too well—when your child is screaming because their toast is cut the "wrong" way, when leaving the playground becomes a public spectacle, or when you're running on three hours of sleep and questioning whether you're cut out for this. But instead of judging or shaming, she offers insight. Instead of guilt, she offers grace.

Most importantly, Devon offers hope. Her message that "toddlerhood doesn't have to be terrible" isn't just wishful thinking; it's grounded in solid science and years of experience helping thousands of families transform their daily interactions. When we understand what's happening in our toddler's developing brain and respond with connection, empathy, and developmentally appropriate expectations, these years can become a time of wonder and growth, deepening your relationship with your little one and laying the groundwork for a lifetime of connection.

In fact, the prefrontal cortex—what Dan Siegel and I call the "upstairs brain" in our book *The Whole-Brain Child*—plays a huge role in impulse control, decision-making, empathy, and emotional regulation. It won't be fully developed until they're in their mid- to late twenties, but the experiences they have now play a large role in how that upstairs brain is built and wired. Toddlerhood is a crucial time for building the staircase between their more reactive "downstairs brain," which is already well-developed at birth, and the upstairs brain, which is built from the experiences they have now and throughout childhood. That's not meant to pressure you. It can embolden you to learn ways to be with your toddler that cultivate their development and help you elicit the cooperation that allows you and your toddler to find rhythms that work for both of you.

With that in mind, this book is a bridge—from chaos to clarity, from control to connection, from outdated discipline to developmentally appropriate guidance. Devon is helping to shift generational patterns by inviting parents to bring curiosity instead of criticism, collaboration instead of coercion. She's helping parents break cycles of disconnection and unrealistic expectations and write a new story for their families: one rooted in empathy, regulation, and secure attachment.

This is why this work matters. Because how we respond in these ordinary, messy moments shapes our child's nervous system. It forms the foundation for how they will understand safety, trust, and self-worth. It builds their actual brains. And it shapes us too. Toddlerhood, when met with intention and reflection, has the power to grow not just resilient kids, but resilient parents.

As you dive in, remember that both you and your toddler are learning and growing together. You don't have to get it right all the time. The strategies you'll discover here won't eliminate all challenging behaviors. That would be impossible. Instead, they'll help you become the (more) calm, confident guide your child needs as they navigate this remarkable time. You'll learn to see meltdowns as windows into your child's inner world and nervous system, defiance as a healthy sign of growing independence, and those exhausting daily moments as opportunities to build lifelong skills.

If you're a parent who has ever felt like you were failing because your toddler wouldn't listen, or like you've lost yourself in the process of trying to stay calm through back-to-back meltdowns, this book will feel like a lifeline. Because when you know differently, you show up differently—and then everything changes. As you find yourself more effective in navigating the hard stuff, you'll have more bandwidth to play, to have fun, and to delight in your child.

Read it. Savor it. Let it challenge you, comfort you, change you, and support you as you're doing the most important job in the universe: nurturing the heart, mind, and brain of your child.

All the best to you,

Tina Payne Bryson, PhD
Coauthor of *The Whole-Brain Child*, *No-Drama Discipline*, *The Yes Brain*, *The Power of Showing Up*, and *The Way of Play*; author of *The Bottom Line for Baby*

Introduction

THE TRUTH ABOUT TODDLERHOOD

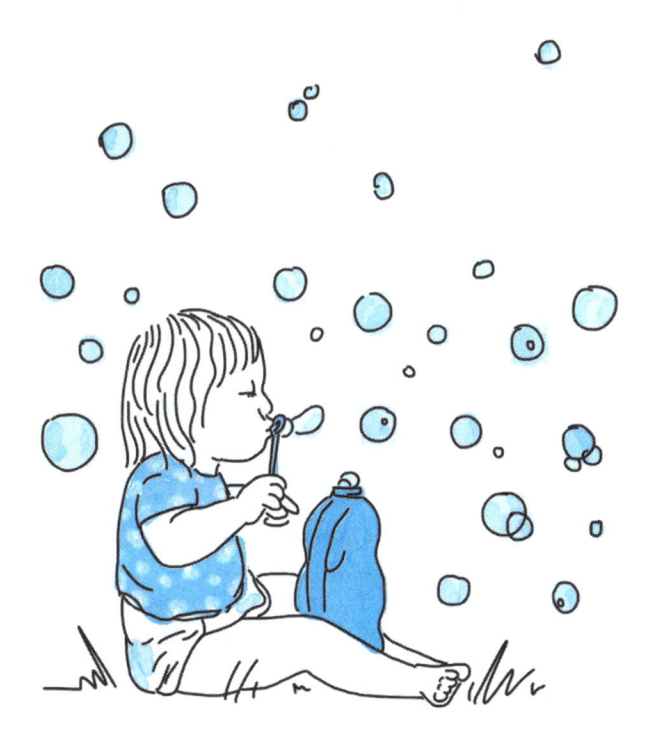

Chapter 1

WELCOME TO TRANSFORMING TODDLERHOOD

Parenting is hard.

No, scratch that.

Parenting can feel like just barely surviving on a *good* day—especially when you're the parent or caregiver of a toddler. Your shirt is stained with some unknown substance. You look around your house and see toys, dishes, and laundry piled up higher than the New York City skyline. Showering? Ha! Might as well be a luxury spa vacation. And you're already exhausted before the sun has risen. The first hour of your day may look something like this:

> 5:30 a.m.: Your toddler is up and so is the household.
> 5:46 a.m.: The amount of effort it takes to convince your toddler to change out of their beloved puppy pajamas is akin to negotiating a peace treaty.
> 5:55 a.m.: The seemingly innocent question "What do you want for breakfast?" opens Pandora's box.
> 6:00 a.m.: You decide to put the cereal in the *Bluey* bowl. It's the wrong choice. The world might end if your beloved toddler does not receive their cereal in the *PAW Patrol* bowl.

6:02 a.m.: Hold up, they don't want cereal anymore! *Why did I even offer cereal?!* you wonder as the meltdown commences.

6:14 a.m.: Oh wait, they *do* want cereal—as long as it has milk.

6:15 a.m.: Now that the milk has been added, your toddler needs a spoon. But not the green spoon. Anything but the *green* spoon!

And folks, that's all before you've even had a chance to take a single sip of coffee. An average day for parents of toddlers is a whirlwind of big emotions and never-ending tasks. You wake up tired from a night of interrupted sleep, brace yourself for morning tantrums about breakfast and power struggles about getting dressed, and proceed to navigate the day trying to keep your child engaged and "out of trouble" (all the while trying to maintain the things you did before having children) *aaand* attempting to stay calm in the process.

The emotional highs and lows and the physical demands are exhausting, and by the end of the day, many parents feel drained and defeated. Of course, you want to enjoy this precious time with your child, but you find yourself caught in a cycle of power struggles and tantrums that leave you feeling burned out and maybe even resenting your child instead.

Raising a toddler can be grueling and challenging, but it's also a pivotal time in your child's life—and in your own.

The reality? You're going to make mistakes, you're going to lose your temper, and at times, you might even resort to coercive, fear-based parenting. But this doesn't mean you're a bad parent. You're not failing. You, just like your little one, are a human, and that means you're both works in progress and still learning.

What you need is more support and better tools to discover a more effective way to navigate this journey of raising a toddler.

Don't Tame, *Transform*

In the early days of my career, I worked as a nanny for high-profile families across the globe—and trust me, I've seen it *all* when it comes to toddler behaviors. The crying. The tantrums. The power struggles.

One day stands out vividly in my memory.

Three-year-old Henry was in rare form. From the moment he woke up, it seemed like everything was a trigger for a meltdown. His breakfast was too hot, his favorite shirt was in the wash, and his toy car wasn't zooming the way he wanted it to. By midmorning, he was in full meltdown mode—screaming, hitting, kicking, biting, slapping, and breaking things. I felt my heart sink as I watched this small, furious tornado destroy everything in his path.

I tried everything I could think of to tame this wild behavior. I offered him his favorite snacks, tried to distract him with songs, and even attempted to give him a hug. When that didn't work, I put him in time-out—repeatedly—but that would only make him kick and scream *more*. Each attempt to control his behavior seemed to escalate his frustration. And the more frustrated and dysregulated he became, the more frustrated and dysregulated I became.

Here I was, a professional with a degree in psychology, years of experience, and a wealth of knowledge in child development, and I couldn't calm this tiny, enraged human. I sank to the floor, feeling like an absolute failure, completely desperate, and increasingly infuriated all at the same time. That's when the tears started flowing.

Sitting on the floor of that living room amid the wreckage of toys (and a broken lamp), I knew things had to change. We couldn't go on like this!

Then it hit me: I'd been measuring my success by his behavior. Every tantrum, every power struggle, every "bad" moment felt like a personal failure. But suddenly, I realized—his behavior wasn't "bad," and I wasn't a "failure" when things spiraled. I had been so wrapped up in stopping the outbursts and getting him to obey, so focused on "fixing" his behavior, that I lost sight of what really mattered: our relationship. It was clear that we saw each other as opposing forces and most definitely not as teammates trying to work together. And in that moment, I understood that true progress starts with prioritizing that connection over perfect behavior.

Spoiler alert: Prioritizing compliance over connection won't work—especially in the long term.

So I began making a shift. I started to see the behavior as a form of communication. Henry wasn't trying to be difficult; *he was trying to tell me something*. He was overwhelmed! Frustrated! And unable to articulate his feelings in a way that made sense to him. I needed to reframe my perspective. Instead of trying to tame the behavior, I needed to *transform* my approach. This wasn't about exerting control; it was about being in charge. I needed to disarm my triggers, understand the needs driving Henry's behavior, and respond with empathy and connection while still setting clear limits and helping him follow through.

With this new mindset, I began to see changes. Instead of reacting to Henry's outbursts with frustration, I responded with calmness and empathy. I learned to recognize the emotions and needs behind his behavior. I acknowledged his feelings, helped him find words to express himself, and set clear, consistent limits. I focused on teaching him skills to manage his emotions rather than simply trying to stop the outbursts. It was a process—one that didn't happen overnight and that I didn't do perfectly—but slowly, our days became more peaceful and joyful.

And let's be clear: Henry didn't stop acting like a toddler (I mean, tantrums are a part of the gig!), but I began to understand his behavior on a deeper level and learned how to respond to it in an effective, developmentally appropriate way. It wasn't all rainbows and butterflies, but I did feel more confident, calm, and capable of handling whatever challenge came my way.

Inspired by the success of this approach, I wanted to share what I had learned with others. I realized that many (read: *all*) parents and caregivers struggled with the same issues I had faced, and I wanted to help them find the same sense of confidence and joy I had discovered, especially now as a mama. And so, Transforming Toddlerhood was born.

Through Transforming Toddlerhood, I educate a community of more than one million parents and caregivers from around the world, providing them with tools and strategies to overcome the chaos of toddlerhood, and, most importantly, to nurture their children's development and joyfully experience this precious time. Transforming Toddlerhood is more than just a business or a community—it's a mission to change the way we approach parenting young children during a critical developmental period.

WELCOME TO TRANSFORMING TODDLERHOOD

The Goal of *Transforming Toddlerhood*

Toddlers are *not* terrible. Yet parenting toddlers comes with a myriad of challenges. On the inside, parents often feel overwhelmed and frustrated, struggling with self-doubt and guilt, wondering if they're doing enough or if they're doing it right. On the outside, they face the relentless demands of a toddler's emotional and physical needs, the societal pressure to have a "well-behaved" child, and the constant juggle of balancing parenting with other responsibilities.

Which is why the goal of *Transforming Toddlerhood* is simple: to make this critical yet challenging developmental period easier so you can nurture your child's development, raise an emotionally healthy child, and be the parent you always envisioned. This transformation is about moving from control to connection, from frustration to understanding, and from power struggles to cooperation.

In this book, we'll answer the questions you may be asking yourself: *Where's this (behavior) coming from? What is my child really trying to tell me? How can I keep myself calm? How can I respond in a way that will support their development and help this go smoother next time? How can I calm the chaos instead of adding to it?*

This is what's possible when parenting is rooted in connection and developmentally appropriate expectations. Imagine what it would feel like if you were able to

- start each day with confidence in your parenting approach, knowing you have the tools to handle whatever the day brings;
- stay calm no matter how your child behaves, turning challenging behavior into moments of connection rather than conflict;
- prevent and transform challenging behaviors using effective tools that don't leave you feeling guilty;
- handle power struggles with patience and clarity, transforming moments of defiance into opportunities for growth;
- internalize the truth that you don't have to be a perfect parent—just a present one who learns and grows alongside their child; and

- spend more time enjoying parenting and having fun with your child instead of fighting a constant battle that leaves you mentally and emotionally drained.

By embracing the principles outlined in this book, you'll transform not only your child's behavior but also your own experience of parenting. You'll move from feeling like you're barely surviving as a family to truly thriving and connecting with one another.

Ready? Let's transform.

THREE GOALS OF THIS BOOK

1. Gain a deeper understanding of toddler development and how it impacts behavior.
2. Learn effective, developmentally appropriate tools and skills for responding to challenging behaviors.
3. Discover ways to make parenting easier so you can fully enjoy this critical and magical stage of development.

Chapter 2

WHAT IS A TODDLER AND HOW DO YOU KNOW YOU HAVE ONE?

When your little one was a baby, mornings began slowly—soft whimpers inviting you to scoop them up, their tiny body snuggling into yours as you rocked them. You could linger in those quiet moments, breathing in their smell and marveling at their peaceful, squishy face.

But today? Today is another story. There's no gentle cooing. Instead, you hear a thud as little feet hit the floor, followed by the pitter-patter of a determined toddler on a mission. Your once-quiet baby has transformed into a demanding, fast-talking, independent tiny tyrant with a loudspeaker.

Toddlerhood is the stage where they start to figure out that they're their own person, separate from you. They've got their own agenda, and they want it taken seriously. You might be wondering, *What happened to my cuddly baby? How long is this going to last?*

The Shift from Infancy to Toddlerhood

In the baby season, you were your child's everything—their source of soothing, nurturing, and protection. They saw themself as an extension of you, and you often saw them the same way.

But a toddler's world is about exploration, independence, and testing boundaries. That sleepy newborn who once curled up against your chest is now running ahead of you, pushing limits, and showing you, in no uncertain terms, that they are their own person. A toddler is still highly dependent on you to meet their physical and emotional needs, but, at the same time, they are trying to become their own person. Where babies seek closeness, toddlers want autonomy—but they also desperately need comfort and help managing the big emotions they're struggling to understand. This creates a lot of contradictory feelings and needs that toddlers struggle to communicate and navigate.

It's no longer about just keeping them fed and content—you've got to navigate their growing sense of independence while still setting the necessary limits. This is a major shift, and it's easy to start questioning yourself. *What is going on here? Am I doing this right? Why is it so much harder now?!*

Toddlerhood is a whirlwind of learning, growth, and chaos. It's messy, loud, and at times exhausting, but it's also magical. You get to hear your little one talk for the first time and meet their emerging personality. You're no longer simply caring for a baby—you're now guiding a small, fierce person who is discovering the world and their place in it. You've leveled up, and while the challenges are different, the rewards are even greater. Welcome to the toddler years.

What Is a Toddler?

Toddlerhood begins as early as nine to fifteen months and ends at your child's fifth birthday. The term *toddler* comes from the moment your child starts to toddle—those shaky first steps that mark their budding independence. But toddlerhood isn't just about walking. It's a whole developmental phase where your little one is learning, for the very first time, who they are and how to navigate the world.

I like to break down toddlerhood into two main phases—younger toddlers and older toddlers—to best understand their development and the shifts that come with it.

Younger Toddlers
(One to Two Years Old)

In the early toddler phase, children primarily use both crying and physical actions to communicate. Your child is learning how to navigate their emotions, and crying is a way for them to communicate their frustration, discomfort, or need—along with hitting, biting, throwing, kicking, screaming, and tantrums—as they figure out how to make themself understood. Though their words may still be limited, they understand more than they can say. By fifteen months, most toddlers can comprehend simple instructions like "Go get your shoes" or "Come here," even if they can't yet verbally respond. Once they reach eighteen months, toddlers understand about two hundred to five hundred words but can say only around fifty.[1] It's important to talk to young toddlers as if they do understand you because their receptive language is growing rapidly, and it's a great time to use baby sign language to support the growth of their expressive language.

Older Toddlers
(Three to Four Years Old)

As your toddler approaches three, you'll likely notice a shift. This season is marked by less crying, fewer outbursts (though tantrums still happen!), and more words. By this stage, your child has developed a more consistent way of expressing their wants and needs through language, but they are still not always able to find the right words to express themself, especially if they are experiencing big emotions or are overstimulated. While tantrums may become less frequent, your toddler's desire for independence and control over their environment continues to grow.

Transitioning from Toddlerhood
(Five Years Old)

By age five, your child is moving beyond toddlerhood, showing greater emotional regulation and a stronger ability to express complex feelings with words, making meltdowns less frequent. Socially, they're learning about fairness, sharing, and empathy, which helps them form deeper friendships and handle group dynamics more easily.

SIGNS YOU'VE ENTERED TODDLERHOOD

- **Saying No:** This is a toddler's way of asserting independence. By saying no, they are testing limits and boundaries, plus learning to be their own person who is separate from you.
- **Hitting, Biting, and Kicking:** These actions are often impulsive responses to frustration or overstimulation. Toddlers lack the verbal skills to express their feelings and may resort to physical actions to communicate.
- **Throwing:** Whether it's a toy or food, throwing objects can be a way for toddlers to explore cause and effect, as well as to express frustration and test which behaviors get a reaction from you.
- **Tantrums:** Meltdowns are common as toddlers experience strong emotions and sensory overwhelm that they do not yet know how to manage. Tantrums are a typical and important part of emotional development and can be a way for children to release pent-up feelings.
- **Running Away:** Toddlers have a natural curiosity and desire to explore their environment. Running away can be a game and a way to assert independence.
- **Limit Testing:** Toddlers are *wired* to test the limits we set. When a toddler looks you in the eye and does the opposite of what you've asked, they are testing boundaries and learning about consequences.
- **Possessiveness:** Toddlers may become possessive of toys, people, or spaces, often declaring "Mine!" as they learn about ownership. This behavior is part of their growing awareness of self and boundaries, helping them establish their sense of identity.
- **Resisting Containment:** Toddlers often resist anything that makes them feel contained, as their growing independence

> drives a need for freedom and movement. This can lead to battles over diaper changes, car seats, high chairs, strollers—anything that restricts their movement and exploration feels like a challenge to their autonomy.

All Behavior Is Communication

These behaviors, while challenging, are *developmentally appropriate*. Toddlers communicate their feelings, emotions, and needs not only through words but also through their *behavior*. Behavioral communication is not a sign of a "bad" child but rather an indicator that a toddler is learning and growing. Take saying no, for example: The constant no is a crucial part of developing a sense of self! This phase is about toddlers beginning to understand that they are separate individuals with their own thoughts and desires. By understanding and reframing toddler behaviors, we can shift our perspective from frustration to understanding and navigate common challenges more effectively.

Toddlerhood is a time of enormous growth—physically, emotionally, socially, and cognitively. In this process, it's important to remember that behaviors we may find challenging are often part of a toddler's natural development.

The toddler years are when your little one starts to step into their own personality and begins to discover their preferences, boundaries, and desires. Yes, it can be challenging to keep up with their ever-changing moods and contradictory needs, but it's also a magical time when they're learning about the world at lightning speed, and we start to learn who they are as an individual.

If you've ever found yourself negotiating over snack choices, racing to put on a diaper before they wriggle away, or navigating a meltdown over which cup is acceptable today—you, my friend, have a toddler.

TODDLER LIKES AND DISLIKES

Likes	Dislikes
showing affection on their own terms	sitting still, especially at mealtimes
testing limits	being restrained, especially in car seats or for diaper changes
moving their bodies	being told what to do
touching and exploring everything	having their play interrupted
doing things on their own	going to sleep on their own
being in charge of their bodies	sharing with others
reading the same books over and over again	being separated from their parents
following you everywhere	changes in routine
being held	brushing their teeth and getting dressed

Chapter 3

TODDLERS AREN'T TERRIBLE

Toddlerhood has a pretty lousy PR team. Society has coined plenty of terms to describe this stage—*threenagers, fierce fours, tiny tyrants*. By the time your baby's first birthday rolls around, whispers of the impending "terrible twos" haunt you like a spoiler alert you didn't ask for. Well-meaning friends, family, and even strangers at the grocery store will warn you that toddlers are out to manipulate you, painting this phase as an emotional storm, a relentless battle between their defiance and your sanity.

It's easy to understand why the labels have stuck: Toddlers are swiftly gaining *physical* independence yet are still extremely *emotionally* dependent on us, ready to push limits but without the brain maturation and life experience to have self-control. These competing needs lead to conflict—cue the tantrums, refusals, and power struggles. But labeling an entire developmental period as "terrible" does a disservice to the beauty of your child's development and your role in nurturing them while being an effective parent.

Can toddlerhood *feel* terrible during a grocery store meltdown? Absolutely.

But are toddlers themselves inherently terrible or bad?

No! In fact, *there is no such thing as a terrible toddler*!

When we get stuck on the "terrible" label, we miss out on the chance to embrace one of the most profound, accelerated learning periods in a human being's life. Accepting these labels disempowers us as parents, feeding a cycle of negativity that can make toddlerhood harder than it needs to be. How you approach this critical developmental period will shape not only the way you experience your child but also their behavior.

When we remind ourselves that toddlers have hardly *any* life experience and that their brains are undergoing massive development, it helps to reframe our own narrative. They are looking to us for guidance in every moment, even when it seems like they are pushing you away or trying to push your buttons on purpose. They're taking a crash course in humanhood—emotions, relationships, problem-solving—and you're not just along for the ride; you're their guide.

The truth about toddlerhood? Yes, it can be challenging, but it's also a foundational period that sets the stage for the rest of your child's life. Every day, your child is growing, learning, and changing, making this one of the most exciting phases of development. And those "terrible" moments? Those are visible signs of all the unseen work happening in your child's brain. It's not about your toddler being terrible; it's about their world growing more complex by the day and their attempts to find their footing. It's tough being a toddler parent—and it's also tough being a toddler.

COMMON MYTHS ABOUT TODDLERHOOD

Myth #1: Toddlerhood is terrible.

Reframe: Toddlerhood is a critical developmental period that can feel challenging. Toddlers are becoming their own people and developing a sense of self for the very first time. As a result, behaviors like saying no, testing limits, and throwing tantrums are a typical part of toddlerhood that can leave parents feeling frustrated.

Myth #2: Toddlers are being bad when they act out.
Reframe: Toddlers are having a hard time when they have behavior we find challenging. Toddlers communicate their feelings, emotions, and needs the best way they know how—often with their behavior.

Myth #3: Toddlers are manipulative.
Reframe: Toddlers are strategic in getting their needs and wants met. They are exploring their influence on the world around them and testing boundaries to understand cause and effect, not to manipulate outcomes.

Myth #4: Toddlers should be able to control their emotions and behavior.
Reframe: Toddlers are not capable of controlling their emotions (and, consequently, their behavior) consistently. Expecting toddlers to have adultlike emotional and behavior regulation ignores their lack of brain maturity, where impulse control is still developing. They're learning to manage their emotions gradually, with caregivers playing a crucial role in modeling and guiding them through emotional expression and regulation.

Myth #5: Toddlers should listen the first time.
Reframe: Toddlers are *not* capable of listening the first time. The belief that toddlers should immediately comply with directives overlooks their developmental wiring. They are their own people, developmentally wired to exert their will and explore their environment.

Amid the endless messes, sleepless nights, and temper tantrums, it's easy for us parents to lose sight of the beauty and wonder that defines this phase of childhood. Yet, within the chaos, there are countless reasons to embrace and cherish toddlerhood—not just for our children's sake but for our own growth and learning as well.

Reasons to Love the Toddler Years

Look, I get it. When you're sleep-deprived and just trying to keep everything on track, it's hard to remember the magic of these early years. But our brains tend to notice what we focus on. Therefore, you may need a gentle nudge to shift your focus to the positive and fun aspects of toddlerhood. This simple change can completely transform your experience and build your resilience for the tough moments.

- **Exciting Firsts:** The toddler years are a time of unparalleled discovery. This season is a series of "firsts"—the first tentative steps as they learn to walk, the first triumphant ride on a tiny bicycle, the first independent use of the potty, and those precious first words. Each milestone is a celebration of growth, a testament to resilience, and a reminder of the sheer joy that comes from witnessing the world through fresh eyes.
- **Unconditional Love:** In the world of toddlers, love is unconditional and boundless. They love fiercely, without hesitation or reservation. Their hugs are tight, their smiles infectious, and their ability to forgive and forget is a lesson in grace. As parents, we learn from them the profound capacity to love without expecting anything in return, to embrace vulnerability, and to nurture relationships with openness and warmth.
- **Living in the Moment:** Toddlers live fully immersed in the present, oblivious to past regrets or future worries. They can be mad at you one moment and the next moment be happily playing like nothing ever happened. They teach us to slow down, let go of the past, and appreciate the beauty of the present without holding a grudge.
- **A Desire to Learn:** For toddlers, learning is not a chore but a joyful journey of discovery. They eagerly soak up knowledge through play, turning every moment into an opportunity to learn and grow.

Their boundless enthusiasm for new experiences inspires us to approach challenges with a sense of playfulness and to embrace lifelong learning as a source of joy.

- **Full-Stop Honesty:** Toddlers have no filter when it comes to honesty. Whether commenting on the appearance of a stranger or declaring their distaste for peas at the dinner table, their unabashed honesty can be refreshing. They teach us the importance of authenticity, of speaking our truth with courage and kindness, and of embracing vulnerability in our relationships.
- **Joy in Small Things:** To a toddler, joy can be found in the simplest of pleasures—a butterfly flitting by, a puddle to splash in, or a cardboard box transformed into a spaceship. In their world, each moment is an opportunity for discovery and delight. They remind us that happiness is often found in moments of pure simplicity and that life's greatest treasures are often hidden in plain sight.
- **Unapologetically Authentic:** Perhaps most importantly, toddlers are unashamed of being themselves. They dance with abandon, sing at the top of their lungs, wear their emotions on their sleeves, and paint with wild strokes outside the lines (and sometimes on the rug). They remind us of the value of self-acceptance, of embracing our flaws and quirks, and of living authentically without the fear of judgment.

> For a printable PDF to hang up as a reminder when the going gets tough, visit transformingtoddlerhood.com/bookresources.

Parenting your toddler isn't about who has the least number of tantrums, the easiest bedtime, or the healthiest of snacks. The journey looks different for everyone, and that's okay. Comparing your toddler's behavior to the behavior of others undermines their individual journey and unique developmental pace.

You have a choice. You can wish this challenging phase of toddlerhood away, repeating the same ineffective tools and hoping things change, or you can fully embrace this developmental stage, equipping yourself with effective tools and skills to nurture your child by being their guide. This is your invitation. Yes, it can be tough (really tough), and it won't look perfect. It requires a willingness to learn, to make mistakes, to learn from those mistakes, and to keep trying. There will be days when you want to throw in the towel, but trust me: A few years from now, you'll look back and feel grateful you embraced the journey with all its ups and downs, its laughter, wonder, and pure joy.

My hope is that by seeing the beauty of toddlerhood, we not only nurture our children's growth but also rediscover ourselves—learning, growing, and finding joy in the magical chaos of this phase of life.

Chapter 4

HOW TO USE THIS BOOK

When you're in the eye of the toddler hurricane—covered in pasta sauce, broken sound barriers, and teeth marks—the last thing you want is a complicated treasure hunt searching for clues and answers to your very real (and very immediate) issue at hand. That's why I have written this book with forty-five short, digestible, easy-to-implement-*right-now* chapters.

What This Book Is and Isn't

Think of this book as your trusted, on-call best friend ready to offer guidance and support whenever you need it. Kid throwing spaghetti at the wall to see if it sticks? Turn to chapter 35. Not brushing their teeth . . . again? Your answer awaits in chapter 33. Can't get them to snooze? Chapter 32 has you covered. Catch them in a lie? Bam, chapter 39. Is there a new baby on the way and you're nervous about Kid 1 meeting Kid 2? Chapter 45 has your back.

Every parent wishes their kid came with a manual—this book is as close as it gets. But let's be clear: This isn't a book of shortcuts. You can't hack your way through nurturing your child's physical, cognitive, and emotional development, or through teaching them skills, building partnership, or fostering real connection. And there's certainly no shortcut to setting clear, kind, developmentally appropriate limits—and actually following through on them.

There's no one-size-fits-all guide to toddlerhood because every child is unique. What works for one family might not work for another—and that's okay! Thriving is not about finding the "right" way to parent; it's about figuring out what works for you and your child. Some children take longer to warm up than others. Some will happily eat their veggies; others reject anything green. Some have learned how to use the potty by age two; others are still working on it at age four. All of this is normal, and accepting that each child's journey unfolds differently is the first step toward a more flexible and joyful approach to parenting. The key is embracing the individuality of your child and the unique path your family is on and recognizing that progress comes with patience and persistence.

As you dive into this book, remember: *Progress takes practice*, and it's how we handle the ups and downs that matters. Even small wins are wins! Take it day by day, and don't be hard on yourself (or your child) if one day doesn't go as planned. A common mistake is trying a tool or technique once or twice and giving up when it doesn't "work" right away. Keep in mind that your child isn't a robot (and neither are you!). Learning new skills takes time. Focus on one change at a time, try it consistently for a few weeks, and then evaluate how it's working for both you and your child. Small, steady adjustments make all the difference.

With each technique you practice from these pages, you'll start to see parenting less as a source of stress and frustration and more as a source of confidence, growth, and joy. The path may not always be easy and linear, but it's a powerful one—and with each intentional choice you make, you're shaping a brighter future for both you and your little one.

Practical Tools and Insights

To make the content as actionable as possible, in this book, you'll find the following special features:

- **Red Flags:** Potential issues that you can learn to recognize early and address before they escalate.
- **Toddler Tips:** Handy tips designed to help you overcome everyday parenting challenges.
- **Scripts for Communication:** Exact phrases and approaches for how to communicate and respond to your toddler effectively. These are a starting place—*not* the only way to respond.
- **FAQs:** The most frequently asked questions I get from parents with quick and easy-to-implement answers.

For links to specific products and my preferred brands, visit transformingtoddlerhood.com/bookresources.

Navigating the Book

To make it easy for you to find the information you need, the book is divided into five parts. Each part addresses different aspects of parenting and the unique challenges that come with this stage of your child's development. Here's what you can expect in each section.

PART 1: The Toddler Parent

Understand your role as a parent and recognize the importance of taking care of your own well-being.

Being a toddler parent is *hard*—especially when you are faced with a miniature version of yourself and your own childhood starts to resurface. In part 1, we'll lay the foundation, inviting you to consider the type of parent you want to be for your toddler. We'll explore varying parenting roles and learn how to recognize and transform your triggers, how to parent with a partner (even if you don't agree!), and why it's important to prioritize your self-care and mental health in this journey.

PART 2: The Toddler Explained
Gain insights into the development of toddlers and what drives their behavior.

When people hear the word *toddler*, it often conjures up thoughts of "the terrible twos" and torrential tantrums. There are frustrations about toddlers not listening, not eating vegetables, not sleeping, not allowing parents to even go to the bathroom without them in tow. In part 2, we'll dig deep into what drives toddler behavior, how to decode what your child's behavior is telling you, and how to build a foundation of healthy, developmentally appropriate discipline.

PART 3: The Emotional Toddler
Learn techniques for raising an emotionally healthy child and strategies for helping your child manage big emotions effectively.

Big emotions can feel like *a lot* to handle. Often parents feel uncomfortable with or triggered by a child's emotions, and we inadvertently try to shut them down. The truth is you can make the biggest difference in your child's life when they are having the toughest time. It's our job to guide kids through their emotional storm. In part 3, we'll dive into all the emotions, big and small. We'll cover topics ranging from transforming tantrums to calming an upset toddler to disarming power struggles to navigating parental preferences and, perhaps most important, building a child's confidence and self-esteem.

PART 4: The Physical Toddler
Gain tips for navigating bodily autonomy and supporting your child's independence.

Picky eating, bedtime struggles, a refusal to get dressed, fights about brushing teeth, the elusive potty-learning process—these are the classic daily challenges rooted in a toddler's developing bodily autonomy. In part 4, you'll discover how to nurture your child's physical development while learning tools to overcome the most common behavior challenges that parents and caregivers face, including hitting, biting, and picky eating.

PART 5: The Social Toddler
Uncover strategies for raising a child who interacts and communicates effectively with others.

Toddlers don't follow adult social norms and are unabashedly open with their thoughts and feelings. While it can be overwhelming, this isn't a sign of them being rude or selfish; it's perfectly normal toddler behavior. At this stage, toddlers are busy soaking up all kinds of social skills through the everyday interactions they have with parents, caregivers, and the world around them. From addressing challenges such as separation anxiety, lying, and shyness to raising a kid who knows how to share, apologize, and help others to navigating conflict, part 5 tackles all things to do with how your toddler interacts with people.

My hope is that this book becomes a valuable resource for you as you navigate the ups and downs of parenting. Remember, it is here to be used in whatever way works best for you—whether that means reading it cover to cover or dipping into specific sections as needed. My aim is to help you find more confidence in your parenting journey, equipped with the tools to nurture your child's development and find joy in these fleeting yet critical years.

Part 1

THE TODDLER PARENT

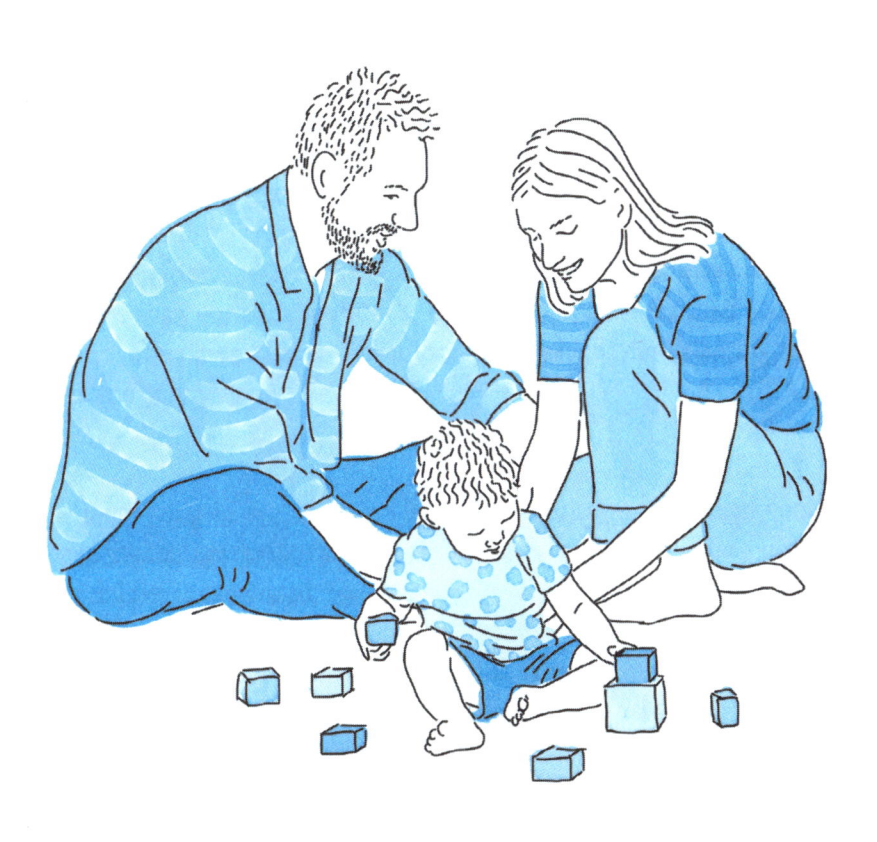

Chapter 5

ESTABLISHING POSITIVE, EFFECTIVE, DEVELOPMENTALLY APPROPRIATE PARENTING

Your toddler, bright-eyed and full of energy, has just refused to leave the playground for the third time. You're tired. Dinner still needs to be made, and you can feel the weight of responsibility pressing down on you. In that moment, it's easy to hear the echoes of generations past:

"If you don't come now, we're never coming back!"

"Fine! I'm going home without you. You can stay here by yourself."

And before you know it . . . the words escape your lips. You hadn't even realized you were going to say them, but your response is rooted in a sense of urgency, frustration, and, yes, fear. These familiar tactics, passed down from well-meaning ancestors, aim to control through threats and punishments, banking on the idea that a child's fear will spur them into obedience.

First of all, when this occurs know this: *You are not a bad parent.* Many of us grew up in homes where conventional, fear-based, and compliance-centered parenting ruled the day—lecturing, punishment, time-outs, and yelling were standard, coercive tools aimed at securing immediate obedience, often at the expense of emotional safety and considering a child's needs.

These go-tos are quick, familiar, and usually create the desired short-term response in kids with more docile personalities. (For spirited kids, the tactics tend to exacerbate unwanted behavior.) Instead of guiding our children, we hope the threat of something bad—being left behind, losing privileges, or facing our anger—will snap them into line. And for a moment, some children may stop, follow, or obey. But at what cost?

Fear Is Not an Effective Teacher

The use of fear-based parenting tactics teaches children not to question people, dims their curiosity, and leads them to comply just to please others. A scared child isn't learning self-regulation skills—they're just avoiding getting in trouble. This style of parenting trades long-term emotional safety and regulation skills for immediate results. We inadvertently teach our children that love, acceptance, and belonging are conditional—tied to their behavior, their compliance, and their obedience.

Here are some examples of what this conventional, fear-based, compliance-centered parenting looks like in action:

- setting unrealistic expectations for behavior that are not based on the child's level of development
- expecting a child to comply and follow the rules without taking their emotional and developmental needs into account
- expecting a child to listen the first time and punishing them if they don't
- using parenting tools based on fear and control (including punishments) to create compliance
- prioritizing compliance over meeting a child's needs or considering their point of view
- believing that obedience equals respect
- lacking parental attunement—the ability to be responsive to child signals, understand them, and respond in a manner that is emotionally supportive

These all take a major toll on the parent-child relationship. When parenting is about control, the trust that's so crucial for healthy development begins to erode, and with it, the emotional safety that should be at the heart of every parent-child bond. Eventually, these little ones grow up to be teenagers who rebel, lie, say yes out of fear of upsetting you, or keep secrets because your relationship has been rooted in a dynamic based on fear, not connection.

There is another way—one that shifts from control to collaboration, from fear to guidance, from threats to understanding. That's where the real transformation begins.

Enter: A New Kind of Parenting

Positive, effective, developmentally appropriate parenting encourages parents to understand the reasons behind a child's behavior, such as emotions, needs, and developmental stages. This is what I call *developmentally smart parenting*. By fostering connection, setting clear expectations, and teaching skills, this form of parenting promotes a supportive environment where children can learn and thrive.

The advantages extend beyond behavior management. Developmentally snart parenting promotes cooperation, optimizes brain development, and reduces power struggles by aligning parenting strategies with a child's natural growth and development. It fosters self-esteem, encourages effective communication, and lays the groundwork for a resilient parent-child relationship that endures through all stages of life. It's about connection, understanding, and a deep commitment to nurturing a relationship built on *mutual respect*. It starts with respecting your child—not just in big moments, but in the everyday, ordinary ones, even when you don't like their behavior.

However, one common misconception is that positive parenting is the same as *permissiveness*. Unlike permissive parenting, which lacks clear boundaries and gives the child too much power, positive parenting balances compassion with firmness. It involves setting developmentally appropriate expectations and limits, while taking a child's needs and emotions into account. It emphasizes teaching children skills for self-control and guiding their behavior through understanding and compassion rather than punishment.

The following are examples of what developmentally smart parenting looks like in action:

- being curious about the root of the behavior or the reason behind it, including consideration for a child's feelings, emotions, needs, desires, temperament, and level of development
- creating connection and prioritizing relationship while still having clear boundaries and limits
- being in control of your words and actions instead of trying to control your child
- teaching tools and skills instead of punishing developmentally appropriate behavior
- looking for what's working and building on the behaviors you want to see with positive reinforcement
- creating clear, developmentally appropriate expectations instead of expecting blind obedience
- focusing on being in charge instead of being in control

POSITIVE, EFFECTIVE, DEVELOPMENTALLY APPROPRIATE RESPONSES

Here are a few examples of intentional responses to common challenges without being permissive:
- Instead of telling your child he is a "bad boy" or "not nice" for hitting, tell him, "That was upsetting, and I won't let you hit. Hitting hurts." Then show him what to do instead.
- Instead of yelling at your child from across the room to stop pulling the dog's tail, help her meet the limit you set by moving her away from the dog.

> - Instead of forcing your child to apologize (or hug a relative), show your child what an apology (or a greeting) looks like. This respects their feelings and boundaries while teaching skills.

Let's revisit that day at the playground.

Your toddler, bright-eyed and full of energy, has just refused to leave the playground for the third time. You're tired. Dinner still needs to be made, and you can feel the weight of responsibility pressing down on you. But instead of falling into the cycle of frustration, ultimatums, or threats, you pause. You take a deep breath, grounding yourself in the knowledge that power struggles don't have to define this moment.

You walk over to your child, crouching down to meet their gaze, and say, "You're having so much fun and don't want to leave. It's hard to stop when you're enjoying something, isn't it?" After a pause, you continue, "It's time to go home. What should we play at home?" Then, you validate their response. "That sounds like fun! Do you want to walk to the car or have Mommy carry you?"

Instead of relying on fear or punishment, you've offered your child a sense of autonomy within the limit you've set. You acknowledged their feelings, creating a moment of connection, and invited them into the process. As a result, they feel seen, heard, and respected—and they begin to learn that transitions don't have to feel like losing control. You're teaching them that cooperation is built on trust, not fear, and it opens the door for smoother transitions, even when you're both tired and stretched thin.

You still might have to carry your child to the car if they refuse to leave, and there might be some tears. But after a few times of you following through on the limits you set, they will know you're serious and stop testing the limit.

Positive, effective, developmentally appropriate parenting isn't just about your kids' growth—it's about growing *together*, building a bond that lasts a lifetime. By keeping it real with positive guidance, you're setting the stage for kids who can handle anything life throws their way.

> ### THE RECIPE FOR POSITIVE, EFFECTIVE, DEVELOPMENTALLY APPROPRIATE PARENTING
>
> Positive parenting requires three essential ingredients:
>
> 1. **Creating Connection:** Building a strong, empathetic bond with your child through understanding, curiosity, validation, and playfulness
> 2. **Setting Clear Limits:** Establishing limits with kindness and consistency—and following through on them—creates a secure environment
> 3. **Teaching Skills:** Guiding children toward positive behaviors through teaching, modeling, practicing, and positive reinforcement
>
> We'll explore this recipe further in part 2.

Making the Shift

Do you want a child who constantly looks outside themself for someone else to set the boundaries, manage their behavior, and tell them to fall in line? A child who complies out of fear or to please others? Or do you want a child who feels safe and secure, developing the skills they need to manage their emotions and, in turn, their behavior?

Transitioning from what we used to think about parenting (the conventional fear- and compliance-based parenting) to a more positive, respectful, effective, and developmentally appropriate parenting involves a *huge* paradigm shift—a commitment to connecting rather than controlling and teaching rather than punishing. And while that can require more effort in the beginning, it may be helpful to know that it's simply *more effective* in the long term. It's a learned skill that requires compassion, self-reflection, and practice—especially during the toddler years.

Chapter 6

UNDERSTANDING YOUR PARENTING ROLE

Have you ever taken a moment to truly reflect on your role as a parent? Sure, keeping your child safe and showering them with love are crucial, but what about the more intricate dimensions of parenting and the subtle roles you embody? Many of us step into parenthood either finding ourselves on autopilot, unintentionally echoing the patterns we learned from our own parents, or having the desire to do things differently but not knowing how to gain and implement the tools and skills needed to effectively accomplish that.

This tension between repeating the familiar and striving for something new often leaves us searching for clarity in our parenting approach. To navigate this, it's helpful to view parenting as a *continuum*.

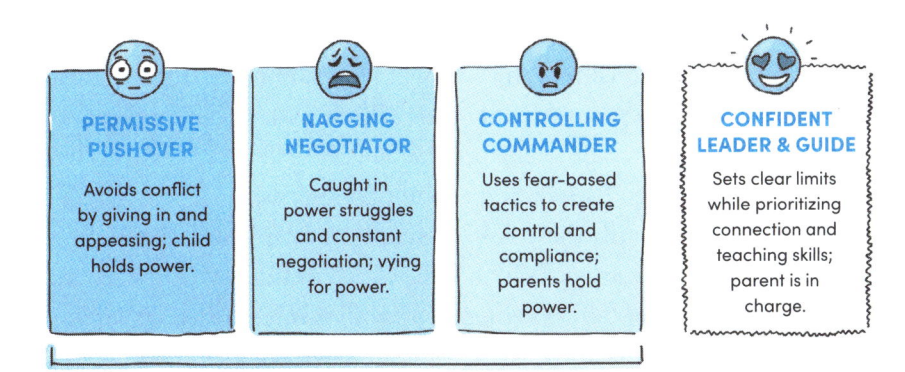

PERMISSIVE PUSHOVER	NAGGING NEGOTIATOR	CONTROLLING COMMANDER	CONFIDENT LEADER & GUIDE
Avoids conflict by giving in and appeasing; child holds power.	Caught in power struggles and constant negotiation; vying for power.	Uses fear-based tactics to create control and compliance; parents hold power.	Sets clear limits while prioritizing connection and teaching skills; parent is in charge.

On one end of the spectrum, we have the **Permissive Pushover**, who tends to set limits but struggles to enforce them. Picture a parent who, with every protest and plea, gives in to the whims of their child, hoping to avoid crying, tantrums, and conflict. This role is defined by an imbalance of power: The child is in control, while the parent becomes a spectator, reacting rather than leading. While this approach might seem to keep the peace in the short term, it often leads to the child having more power than they are developmentally capable of handling, which can make behavior spiral. In this role, the parent feels like they're constantly walking on eggshells, trying to keep the child happy until their boundaries have been crossed too many times and they want to explode.

On the opposite end, there's the **Controlling Commander**, who attempts to dominate and control the child's behavior through yelling, threats, fear, and strict rules. In this dynamic, the parent wields all the power, often dismissing the child's feelings and needs. This role is characterized by an overwhelming sense of authority, where the parent's will is imposed on the child with little regard for the child's feelings or needs. While this method can establish clear rules and order, it risks stifling the child's independence and undermining their emotional well-being. Depending on your child's temperament, they will either comply out of fear or push back to establish independence.

Somewhere in between these extremes lies the **Nagging Negotiator**. This role oscillates between the Permissive Pushover and the Controlling Commander, where the parent and child are locked in a power struggle. In fact, power struggles become the norm. The parent and child are engaged in a constant tug-of-war, each vying for control. The parent's voice is often one of persistent bargaining and pleading, while the child learns to exploit the cracks in this ongoing negotiation to get their needs and desires met. The parent might repeatedly nag, use bribes, or threaten punishment in an attempt to balance the power dynamics, but this often leads to frustration and a lack of meaningful progress.

The challenge with these roles is that they keep you trapped on a disempowering continuum. Whether the child has the power, the parent has the power, or both are vying for it, these dynamics can make parenting extra stressful. It's natural for all of us to move along this continuum from time to time, shifting between roles—but we don't want to make it the norm.

The solution lies in embracing the role of the **Confident Leader and Guide**. This role shifts you off that continuum. Instead of trying to control or compete for power, you step into a place of being in charge. This role represents a balanced approach where authority and empathy coexist. Here, the parent maintains a firm grasp on clear limits while valuing and validating the child's emotions and perspectives. It's a role built on connection, collaboration, and mutual growth. The parent is a guide working with the child to navigate challenges. The power dynamic is no longer a battleground but a nurturing partnership, in which both parent and child contribute to and benefit from the relationship. You create a dynamic where trust and emotional safety are prioritized, alongside clear limits and boundaries.

THE FOUR PARENTING ROLES

Permissive Pushover:
- You set limits but often struggle to enforce them.
- You tend to give in when your child protests with tears or tantrums.
- You may fear your child's emotions, walking on eggshells to avoid upsetting them.
- You strive to keep your child happy at all times, even if it means compromising your own boundaries.

Controlling Commander:
- You attempt to control your child's behavior through yelling, threats, or fear tactics like punishments or spanking.
- You dismiss or ignore your child's feelings and needs.
- You impose strict rules and administer arbitrary consequences for a lack of compliance.

> ### Nagging Negotiator:
> - You and your child have endless power struggles.
> - You find yourself repeating instructions with little result.
> - You resort to threats, bribes, and negotiations to elicit desired behaviors.
>
> ### Confident Leader and Guide:
> - You strive to understand and validate your child's emotions and experiences, ensuring they feel seen and heard.
> - You set and follow through on limits consistently, aiming to teach skills rather than use reactive punishment.
> - You focus on creating win-win solutions where everyone's needs are taken into account.
> - You teach skills and involve your child in problem-solving, fostering a sense of ownership and collaboration.

The goal is to transition away from the disempowered roles of Pushover, Commander, and Negotiator and move toward the empowered role of Leader and Guide. This shift isn't about relinquishing authority but rather about embracing a leadership style that fosters connection, respect, and collaboration while still setting clear limits and boundaries.

Of course, you won't always find yourself perfectly embodying positive, effective, developmentally appropriate parenting as the Confident Leader and Guide (and that's okay!). The goal is to respond *consistently* so it becomes predictable that you will show up as the Confident Leader and Guide more often than not. It takes practice, and there will be moments it feels easy and other moments you want to throw in the towel. It's all part of the journey. Remember, you are already a good parent and your child loves you unconditionally.

The Parenting Roles in Practice

Imagine you're standing near your front door. It's a frigid winter day, you and your kiddo have been cooped up all day, and, secretly, you're dying for a latte. You've got one mission standing between you and your latte: Get the kid into the coat and out the door.

Option 1: The Permissive Pushover

You hold up the coat, but your voice is soft, almost pleading. "Come on, time to put on your coat. It's cold outside."

The response is familiar. "No, I don't want to!"

"But you'll get cold!" You can see what's coming a mile away. "Just put it on, please?"

"Noooo! *I don't want to!*"

With a resigned sigh, you concede. "Okay, fine, we'll just go without the coat then."

Your toddler cheerfully heads out, and you follow, bracing yourself against the biting wind. As they shiver, you watch, knowing you've let the limit slip but feeling too weary to enforce it now.

Option 2: The Controlling Commander

You take a deep breath and channel the drill sergeant within you. With the coat in hand, you command, "Okay, put on your coat. Now." Your tone is firm, unyielding. There's no room for discussion—this is an order.

Their face scrunches up in defiance. "No, I don't want to!"

Without missing a beat, you grab their arms, forcing one and then another through the sleeves. They squirm and wriggle, but you're resolute. The coat is on, and you march outside, filled with a sense of victory and a touch of guilt because your toddler is upset and you feel like a mean parent. The warmth of your bond feels like it's been left at the door.

Option 3: The Nagging Negotiator

Holding out the coat with a hopeful smile, you say, "All right, come on, you need to put your coat on. It's cold outside."

They, per usual, resist. "No, I don't want to!"

"But you'll get cold! Just put it on, please?"

"No, I don't want to!"

"I'll get you a cake pop at the coffee shop if you just put it on! Pretty please?!"

"No!"

"Okay, what about a cake pop *and* a hot chocolate?"

Thus begins a battle of constant bargaining and bribing. A tug-of-war. Yes! No! Yes! No! What if *this*? What if *that*? Maybe you make it out the door, maybe not. Either way, you are too exhausted to care!

Option 4: The Confident Leader and Guide

Holding out the coat, you say calmly, "It's time to put on your coat so we can go outside."

They shake their head with a familiar resistance. "No, I don't want to!"

You kneel to their level, hand them the coat, and offer a choice. "I hear you aren't ready to put on your coat. You can hold it if you don't want to put it on right now. Then if you get chilly, you'll have it."

The two of you walk toward the car as they play with the coat, fidgeting with the zipper. Soon, their little body begins to shiver. Your toddler looks up at you, a spark of realization in their eyes. "I want my coat on now!"

With a gentle smile, you guide the little arms into the sleeves. In that moment, you feel a deep sense of accomplishment—not just for avoiding a power struggle by using natural consequences and getting out the door, but for guiding your child with respect and understanding (okay, and maybe because you're actually gonna get that latte you've been craving).

Look, parenting isn't just a series of decisions and actions—it's a dynamic interplay of power and influence, shaped by our roles and relationships with our children. Understanding where we fall on the spectrum of parenting roles can transform not just how we guide our children but how we build lasting, meaningful relationships with them. By moving toward the role of Confident Leader and Guide, you embrace a balanced approach that honors both your authority and your child's autonomy. This role fosters a positive, supportive environment where both you and your child can thrive.

The Key to Becoming a Confident Leader and Guide: A Growth Mindset

At the heart of effective parenting lies a growth mindset—a belief that abilities and qualities can be developed through dedication and hard work. Contrasting with a fixed mindset that sees qualities as unchangeable, a growth mindset allows parents to embrace challenges, learn from mistakes, and encourage persistence in their children.

Fixed Mindset	*Growth Mindset*
Views qualities as unchangeable, leading to stagnation and resistance to change.	Believes in the potential for growth and development through effort and perseverance.

Practicing a growth mindset in parenting involves reframing challenges and setbacks. In pursuit of this, we may make some of the following shifts:

- Move from a fixed mindset of "I'm doing this wrong" to a growth mindset of "I'm still learning and it's okay. Next time I will focus on . . ."
- Move from a fixed mindset of "I'm failing because I'm still yelling at my toddler" to a growth mindset of "I can learn to stop yelling."
- Move from a fixed mindset of "This will never change" to a growth mindset of "Practice makes progress."
- Move from a fixed mindset of "I can't take any more" to a growth mindset of "I can do things that are challenging."
- Move from a fixed mindset of "I don't know what to do" to a growth mindset of "It's possible to figure this out, and I can take the next step without fully knowing where we are headed."

Remember, embracing a growth mindset in parenting allows you to focus on the process rather than the outcome and celebrate the small victories along the way. There's no one-size-fits-all approach. It's about finding what works for you and your child and building on those successes. This is your invitation to embrace the messiness, stay grounded in your role as a Confident Leader, and let your relationship with your child be a source of joy and discovery. You're not just shaping their future; you're both growing together. Keep going, keep learning, and trust that you're doing an amazing job.

Chapter 7

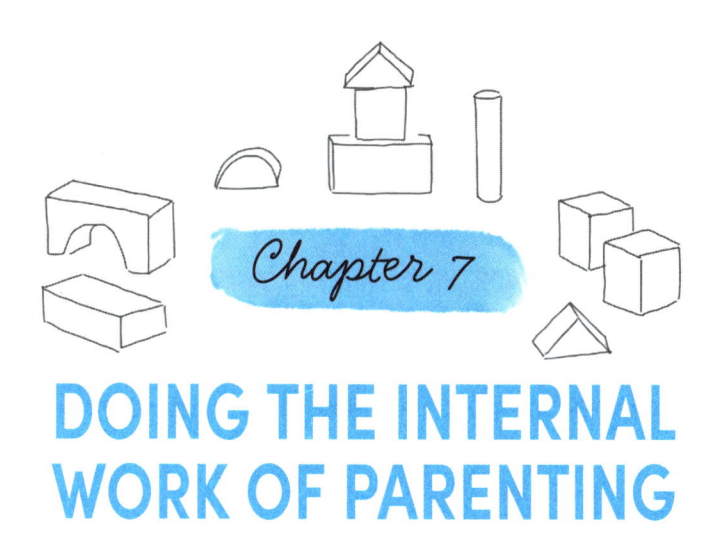

DOING THE INTERNAL WORK OF PARENTING

Parenting toddlers isn't just about managing their big emotions—it's about managing yours. In fact, the hardest part of parenting often isn't the child at all. It's the mirror they hold up to your unresolved wounds, unmet needs, and ingrained patterns.

> **REASONS WHY TODDLERHOOD IS TRIGGERING**
>
> - It makes us face the things that are unresolved within us or that we are still processing from our childhood.
> - This is the first time our parenting skills are tested.
> - It challenges our sense of control.
> - It illuminates unrealistic expectations we hold for what toddlers are capable of developmentally.
> - We're shown we may lack the skills needed to navigate challenging behavior in a positive, respectful, developmentally appropriate way.

Recognizing these triggers is the first step toward breaking generational cycles. The way we react to our children's behavior is often a reflection of how we were parented, and without awareness, we risk repeating patterns we swore we'd leave behind. This is where reparenting comes in—giving ourselves the patience, understanding, and tools we may not have received so we can show up for our children as the Confident Leader and Guide they need.

The Stress Response and Emotional Regulation

Your toddler has been having a tough morning. They're crying and whining at every turn, and you can't figure out why. Maybe they didn't get enough sleep, maybe they are getting sick—who knows! All you know is that it's only seven o'clock and you are already at the end of your rope. Then your toddler bites you when you say they can't watch *Bluey* right now. That's when you lose it and snap at them. You just joined them on their emotional roller coaster. It doesn't feel good, but stopping yourself feels impossible.

To break this cycle, we need to start by looking *inward*. What's really happening in those heated moments? What's going on in your brain when frustration takes over and yelling feels inevitable? Here's the twist—it's the same process happening for your toddler. Let's unpack this together:

- Just like your toddler, when you find yourself yelling or reacting, it's because your brain is doing exactly what it's wired to do in a moment of stress.
- Your **amygdala**, the part of your brain responsible for processing emotions like fear and anger, perceives a threat and kicks the body into emergency mode.
- **Cortisol** floods the system, your heart rate spikes, your breathing quickens, and suddenly, you're in fight, flight, freeze, or fawn mode.

- In these moments, your ability to think clearly, problem-solve, and regulate your emotions diminishes. In other words, you're stuck in **survival mode**, just like your toddler often is.

As adults, our brains are fully mature, and we *still* find it difficult to keep our composure and regulate our emotions and behavior. This emergency response is part of who we all are as humans.

If adult brains can still slip so easily into survival mode, what hope does a toddler who is lacking brain maturation have without our guidance? The good news is, with awareness and intention, we can retrain our responses and model the calm we hope to inspire in our children. (There's more on this in the next chapter.)

Breaking the Cycle of Reactivity

At the root of your stress response is a *trigger*—something that sets off a cascade of feelings. Triggers are the catalyst for creating emotional reactions to specific events or challenges (such as your child's behavior) and often bring you back to a feeling created by a similar past experience. The events or experiences that trigger you can be as obvious as your child's shriek of frustration or as subtle as the tight deadline at work that's been eating at you all day. Triggers often stem from experiences in our own childhoods and how we were raised. Maybe we grew up feeling unheard, powerless, or disrespected. Maybe we internalized the fear of being judged or the need for control.

How to Know If You Are Triggered
- Your response feels automatic, like you can't control it, or it takes you by surprise.
- Your reaction is out of proportion with what's happening.
- Your response includes yelling, shutting down, the desire to punish your child, or feeling angry, upset, or out of control.
- You experience deeper feelings or emotions beneath the surface, such as sadness, disappointment, hurt, worry, or fear.
- You have a strong need to control the situation and your child.

Common Triggers

I feel . . .

unheard	powerless	disrespected	unsafe
judged	blamed	controlled	unloved
excluded	manipulated	helpless	trapped
ignored	uncared for	taken advantage of	not good enough

The reality is that many of us grew up without the tools to express or process the full spectrum of emotions in a healthy way.

So when your child's emotions escalate, and you find yourself yelling—especially if that's how you were parented—it can feel almost impossible to respond differently. But hear this: That is *not* your fault, and it does *not* make you a bad parent.

Change is possible. It takes time, practice, and sometimes the support of a therapist to unpack the past and build a new way forward. There is no shame in that. More than anything, I want you to know: You are not alone.

Reparenting Yourself While Parenting Your Child

One of the things that makes positive, effective, developmentally appropriate discipline so challenging to learn and execute is that it often asks us to reparent ourselves at the same time as we are parenting our children. Your toddler's defiance or meltdowns might feel like personal attacks, but they are developmentally appropriate behaviors, and often they're reflecting back areas where you still need healing. Were you dismissed as a child when you expressed big feelings? Did you grow up in a home where yelling or punishment was the norm? These experiences shape how you react now.

Whether it's whining that grates on your nerves or defiance that makes your blood boil, these triggers aren't random—they're tied to deeper fears or unresolved hurts. Identifying them is the first step toward healing and growing.

Practical Steps for Reparenting

1. **Acknowledge Your Inner Child's Wounds:** Reflect on your childhood and identify moments that shaped your beliefs about emotions, control, or worthiness.
2. **Notice and Validate Your Feelings:** When frustration bubbles up, pause and name it: *I feel unheard right now.*
3. **Practice Compassion:** Remind yourself that you're human—learning and growing, just like your child.
4. **Make Peace with Your Emotions:** Feelings are not good or bad. They make you human. They are valuable signals that can help us understand how we are doing on the inside and tune in to our own unmet needs. Feelings are also temporary. They come and go. Knowing this allows us to accept the full spectrum of emotions we experience without labeling them bad or wrong.
5. **Check with Yourself:** Take a moment each day to ask yourself, *How am I feeling? What do I need right now?*
6. **Seek Support:** Therapy can be a game changer for uncovering, processing, and healing your triggers and childhood wounds plus building new patterns.

Start small and practice. If you have trouble moving the needle, don't get down on yourself. Reach out for support, and always remember: Practice makes progress—*not* perfection.

The goal isn't to become a perfect parent; it's to be a growing one. Every time you pause, every time you repair, every time you choose calm over chaos, you're rewriting the script for both you and your child. You're showing them what it looks like to navigate emotions with grace, even when it's messy.

Parenting is a journey of becoming—becoming the safe parent your child needs and the whole, healed person you deserve to be. Keep going. You're doing the work, and it's worth it.

Chapter 8

BECOMING A SAFE PARENT

I f you've ever yelled at your toddler after a long day or felt frustration surge as they refuse for the fifth time to put on their shoes, take heart—you're not alone. Those moments of yelling or snapping don't define you as a bad parent. You are a good parent who is exhausted, stressed, overwhelmed, and in need of a Calming Plan to create emotional safety. Yes, we all want to yell less, and it's important to work on that. But equally important is what you do *after you yell*—how you repair the relationship. Because the beauty of being human isn't just that we make mistakes; it's that we're capable of learning from them and transforming into the steady, calm presence our children need.

Why Becoming a Safe Parent Matters

A safe parent creates a secure foundation for a child. When children feel physically and emotionally safe, their brains can focus on learning rather than survival. Research shows that constant yelling or punitive discipline like spanking can lead to anxiety, depression, and behavioral issues in children.[1] But when parents prioritize safety—both physical and emotional—parents feel better about themselves and children develop resilience, self-control, and trust.

So what does being a safe parent mean? It means becoming the steady lighthouse in the storm of toddlerhood. A safe parent ensures their child is free from physical harm while also providing the emotional security to express feelings without fear of rejection, shame, or physical reprimands. More specifically, being a safe parent looks like allowing and accepting the full spectrum of emotions without making them bad or wrong, calming yourself first before responding to your child's behavior, and repairing the relationship after yelling.

TODDLER TIP
Repair the Relationship and Make Amends

You tried to stay calm, but your emotions got the best of you and you yelled. Now what?

Step 1: Take Ownership
Own your words and actions by describing what happened.
"I was feeling frustrated, and I yelled."

Step 2: Check In
Check in on how your actions impacted your child and then validate their feelings.
"How did you feel when I yelled? You felt _____. Thanks for telling me."

Step 3: Apologize
Come from a place of empowerment and own it.
"I'm sorry for yelling at you."

Step 4: Create a Redo
Say what you are committed to doing next time and practice it.
"Next time I feel frustrated, I'm going to . . ."

Transform Automatic Reactions into Intentional Responses

When your child's behavior triggers you, the first step is recognizing it—because awareness is the key to breaking the cycle of reactivity. Noticing when tension rises and your body shifts into fight-or-flight mode allows you to step out of automatic reactions and into intentional responses. And this isn't just about avoiding big outbursts—it's about reclaiming your role as the calm, steady presence your child needs.

Reactions are emotions in action. They are raw, unfiltered, knee-jerk responses—words spoken in anger, actions driven by fear, or silence born of overwhelm. While these reactions are natural, they often don't align with the kind of parent you want to be or the family environment you're working to create. The goal isn't to suppress emotions but to separate them from our actions.

It's easy to get stuck in our lower brain, treating everything like an emergency. And while many parenting books and classes emphasize the importance of "pausing before responding," that pause can feel impossible when your body is already in a stress response and your reactions are deeply ingrained. If we truly want to shift from reacting to responding, we must first focus on establishing both **physical and emotional safety**—because only when we feel safe can we create the space to *pause, regulate, and respond with intention*.

Physical Safety
- **Definition:** The degree to which you and your child experience a lack of impending physical harm.
- **Examples:** If your toddler is running toward the road, you do what it takes to stop them. If your toddler bites, you set them down and create some space between you.
- **Why It Matters:** Without physical safety, emotional safety isn't possible because it's hard to disrupt the stress response and calm down when you feel or perceive a potential threat

or emergency. Physical safety creates the space for emotional safety.

Emotional Safety
- **Definition:** The degree to which you can identify, hold space for, and regulate your own emotions, plus hold space for the emotions of your child in a way that is calm and accepting.
- **Examples:** Instead of using positive dismissiveness, as in, "Stop crying! There's no reason to be upset," try, "That's so upsetting. I'm here." Or instead of automatically yelling at your child, work on calming down before addressing their behavior. Instead of "You're making me so mad," try, "I feel frustrated when I ask you to do something and you don't do it."
- **Why It Matters:** Emotional safety builds connection and trust. It shows your child their emotions are not "too much" or "wrong," nor is your child responsible for your emotions.

In the heat of the moment, the first thing to do is remove any real or perceived threats by creating physical safety for your child and yourself.

Once physical safety is established, you can say the five magic words to disrupt the stress response and remove the sense of urgency that causes us to automatically react:

"This is not an emergency."

It's an opportunity to remind yourself that you are safe and your child is safe. I invite you to repeat this out loud. Removing the sense of urgency and disrupting your stress response is the key to pausing so you can intentionally respond.

Why is this so important? Once everyone is safe you can take as much time as you need to calm down. Yes, that means you can address your child's behavior in five minutes or thirty. What matters most is that you disrupt your stress response, come back to your upstairs brain (more on this in chapter 11!), and are able to proceed as a calm, emotionally safe parent. It's vital to calm down *before* moving forward so you can show up as the parent you envision. Here are some of my favorite ways to practice calming down:

Sit or lie down where you are.	Close your eyes.	Breathe in deeply and exhale slowly.	Count (backward, forward, by multiples), timing it with your exhale.
Connect with your five senses.	Back up or leave the room.	Give yourself a hug.	Smell essential oils or light a scented candle that relaxes you.
Acknowledge you are doing your best and so is your child.	Practice EFT, also known as tapping.	Remind yourself that your toddler's behavior isn't about you.	Identify your feeling.

Becoming a safe parent doesn't mean you don't have feelings and emotions. You can't make your feelings and emotions go away. You are not a robot; you are a human being. The more you try to shove down your feelings and emotions, the more likely you are to eventually explode. It's like trying to close the zipper on an overstuffed suitcase. You tug and push until eventually the zipper snaps and the contents go everywhere. What you *can* do is give yourself compassion, keep a growth mindset, and learn to regulate your emotions. You are allowed to learn alongside your toddler. Every time you pause and model calming down, your child is learning.

Creating emotional safety allows us to have a sense of control over the things we can control, such as our own words and actions. It helps rewire our brains to slow down and respond differently to challenging behavior that we may have perceived as a threat in the past. Go slow and steady. Parenting is a marathon, *not* a sprint. Focus on the next step in front of you and it will lead you to the result you are looking for.

Your Calming Plan

Picture this: Your toddler is mid-tantrum, their tiny face flushed with frustration, their voice reaching a decibel you didn't even know was possible. Every fiber of your being is on high alert, ready to react and stop the madness. But deep down, you know that reacting in this moment, in the heat of it all, won't lead you anywhere you want to go. So what do you do?

That's where your **Calming Plan** comes in—a blueprint for breaking the cycle of reactivity and stepping into your power as a parent who responds, not reacts. The Calming Plan adheres to the following three main steps:

1. **Establish Physical Safety:** First things first: Ensure everyone is physically safe. That's priority number one. It's easy to get swept away in the waves of emotions, but before anything else, check that your child, and you, are out of harm's way. This might mean gently guiding them to a softer space or simply taking a step back yourself. Physical safety creates the foundation for everything that follows.

2. **Remove the Urgency:** Take a breath and say those five magic words: "This is not an emergency." When you strip away the urgency, you create space to think, to feel, to be. Urgency is a trickster, making everything feel like a life-and-death situation. But here's the truth: Most of the time, it's not. By reminding yourself that you have time, you give yourself the grace to pause, to gather your thoughts, and to choose your next move wisely.

3. **Create Emotional Safety:** Disrupt your stress response so you can respond in an intentional way. Here are four tools for doing this:
    i. **Calm Yourself:** Practice coming back to your emotional equilibrium. Close your eyes if you can and take a deep breath. Feel your feet on the ground, the air in your lungs. When you're grounded, responding in a calm, emotionally safe way is possible.
    ii. **Shift Your Lens:** Here's where you start to see the bigger picture. Shift your lens from the immediate behavior to what

truly matters: the relationship you're building with your child and the lessons they're learning from you at this very moment. Ask yourself, *What's most important here?* When you focus on the long game, the short-term frustrations start to lose their power. This is your chance to model the kind of behavior you want your child to emulate.

iii. **Take Ownership:** This is where you turn the spotlight inward. Use "I" statements to reflect on your actions and feelings. You might share "I feel frustrated because . . ." or "I need a moment to calm down." Owning your emotions and actions isn't just about taking responsibility; it's about showing your child that it's okay to feel, and it's okay to take a moment to find your center before responding.

iv. **Allow Yourself a Redo:** There will be times when you realize you are yelling or were yelling. It's never too late for a redo. All you have to say is "Whoops! That's not how I want to respond. Let me try again." As you build these muscles your awareness will grow. You will become aware of yelling sooner and sooner until you are aware of the urge to yell before it happens.

Becoming a safe parent doesn't mean having all the answers or never feeling overwhelmed. It's about being the lighthouse, even when the storm is raging inside you and around you.

You won't get it right every time. And that's okay. Don't beat yourself up. You could spend all day in coulda, woulda, shoulda land. That's not productive. Remember the importance of having a growth mindset. Instead of looking through the rearview mirror, look out the windshield toward the future. What matters is that you keep trying, keep practicing. Every time you use this Calming Plan, you're not just managing the moment; you're building resilience, strengthening your bond with your child, and becoming the safe parent you aspire to be.

Hang this plan where you can see it. Let it be a reminder that you have the tools you need to handle whatever comes your way with grace, patience, and love.

Chapter 9

CULTIVATING PATIENCE AND PREVENTING BURNOUT

Before you've even opened your eyes, the mental checklist kicks in. *What's for breakfast? I need to buy swimsuits for the kids before our trip. Running low on diapers—add that to the grocery list. Don't forget to call that client today. And oh, right, snacks for soccer practice—another trip to the store.* It's a never-ending stream, the exhausting mental load of parenting.

Cultivating patience helps you stay present and calm through the ups and downs of toddlerhood, not because you've crossed everything off the list, but because you've found a way to be with what's right in front of you. It's not about doing more; it's about creating room to be the parent you want to be—calm, steady, and fully there in every small, messy, precious moment.

Learning to Set Boundaries

Let's start with the number one most important tool for self-care and preventing burnout: *learning to set boundaries*. Think of boundaries as a protective line around your physical, mental, and emotional well-being. They are deeply personal, shaped by your unique needs and values, and will look different for everyone.

But setting boundaries—especially with children, spouses, extended family, and friends—is anything but easy. You might even feel guilty, as if saying yes to yourself means letting others down. The truth? Boundaries don't make you selfish. They make you stronger. They allow you to preserve your energy, protect your peace, and ultimately show up more fully in your relationships.

Here are some simple yet effective ways to set boundaries in different areas of your life:

- **With Your Child:** "Mommy loves playing with you, and I also need a break. I'm going to sit on the couch for ten minutes [you set a timer], and then I'll be ready to play again."
- **With Your Spouse:** "I need some quiet time to decompress after work before diving into family responsibilities. Let's figure out a plan that works for both of us."
- **With Your In-Laws:** "Dinner at six sounds great! We'll need to leave by seven so we can get the kids to bed on time." "I know Jake's energy can feel overwhelming, but I've got it handled. As his parent, I'll decide how to manage it."
- **With Your Friends:** "That sounds like so much fun! I won't be able to make it this time, but please keep me in mind for next time."

These are just starting points. Like any skill, setting boundaries takes practice, and the more you do it, the easier it becomes. It's okay to say no. It's okay to prioritize your needs. Because when you take care of yourself, you have more to give to those who matter most.

The Default-Parent Dilemma

The default parent is the one who keeps everything together—the master of invisible labor. You know the names of all the teachers, the exact number of frozen waffles left in the freezer, and where every important form is filed without even having to look. You anticipate needs before they arise, juggling tasks so seamlessly that it almost looks effortless—until it's not.

Studies show that default parents often experience chronic fatigue, burnout, and a deep sense of resentment, not just toward their partners but sometimes even toward their children.[1] And perhaps most alarming? That heavy mental load often means you're too worn out to properly take care of yourself, which can really decrease your experience of joy as a parent.

And let's be real: Default parenting is often gendered, with mothers disproportionately bearing the brunt of the mental load. But no matter your gender, carrying the bulk of this labor can feel suffocating. It's easy to fall into the trap of thinking, *If I don't do it, no one will.* This mindset is exhausting, not only because it's true in many cases but also because it breeds resentment.

The antidote? Awareness, communication, and boundaries. Discussing the division of labor with your partner—honestly and openly—can be a game changer. It's about more than just sharing chores; it's about sharing the emotional and mental load that comes with managing a household.

> For more resources on setting boundaries and managing the household as a default parent, visit transformingtoddlerhood.com/bookresources.

THE THREE-STEP PROCESS TO MANAGING OVERWHELM

When the mental to-do list starts to feel like it's written in all caps and neon lights, it's time to pause and take a breath. This simple, three-step process has helped many parents find their way back to calm—to a place where patience can flourish. And I promise, it's doable.

Step 1: Brain Dump

The first step to taming the chaos is simple: Get it all out of your head. Grab a notebook, your phone, a bunch of sticky notes, or whatever works for you, and write down every single task, worry, and reminder swirling around in your mind. Don't try to organize it yet—just let the floodgates open. This brain dump creates space between you and your overwhelm, giving you a clearer perspective on what's really demanding your attention.

Step 2: Sort the List

Once you've got everything on paper, it's time to sort. This is where you start taking back control. Divide your list into three categories:

- **Need:** These are the nonnegotiables, the tasks that absolutely must get done today.
- **Want:** These are the things that would be nice to do if you have the time but won't cause the world to fall apart if they don't happen today.
- **Save for Later:** These tasks can be revisited when you're feeling more grounded, or they can wait for another day entirely.

By breaking down the list, you can focus on what really matters without feeling like you have to do it all at once. It also gives you permission to let go of what can wait.

Step 3: Ask for Support

This might be the hardest part, but it's also the most essential: Ask for help. Whether that looks like asking your partner, a friend, or a family member, or even hiring outside help, it's crucial to recognize that you don't have to do everything alone. Delegate the "want" and "save for later" tasks where you can, and allow yourself to lean on others. This step is not a sign of weakness; it's a sign of strength. Asking for help creates space for you to recharge and prevents the spiral into burnout.

Cultivating Patience Through Self-Care

The key to cultivating more patience? *Take care of yourself.*

If your first instinct is *When do I have the time to focus on myself?* then I'm talking directly to you. Self-care is *critical*. When you're in the trenches of parenting, self-care can feel like a luxury, something you'll get around to once the to-do list is done. But self-care is more than a pedicure or a glass of wine—and it isn't an indulgence. It's the fuel that keeps you going. It's not about pampering yourself for the sake of it but about replenishing your energy so you can show up for your child and yourself with patience, presence, and a full heart.

Think of yourself as a car running on gas. You wouldn't expect to get far on an empty tank, would you? Parenting is the same. If you're running on fumes, trying to power through without taking care of your own needs, you'll eventually break down—physically, emotionally, or both. You can't pour from an empty cup, and self-care is what fills you up.

When you read the words *self-care*, what comes to mind? A spa day? A luxurious bubble bath? These things are great, but really, who has the time for that on a regular basis? The good news is self-care isn't just about grand gestures. In fact, it's more effective when it's woven into your daily routine in simple, accessible ways. Even five minutes can make a huge difference.

Self-care can be approached through different lenses, each addressing unique aspects of well-being. Integrating a variety of self-care types into your routine allows for a more balanced, fulfilling experience, helping you sustain energy, resilience, and, most importantly, patience. Here's a closer look at each type.

Mental Self-Care

Mental self-care is all about nurturing your mind and protecting your mental health. This could mean setting aside time for quiet reflection and managing stress. By taking care of your mental space, you're giving yourself permission to unwind, clear your mind, and recharge.

Examples: Reading a motivational quote each morning, listening to a podcast that uplifts you, journaling, or practicing mindfulness techniques to help reduce mental clutter and keep you grounded.

Emotional Self-Care

Emotional self-care is about acknowledging and honoring your feelings. It involves taking steps to understand your emotions, working through challenging ones, and building a foundation of emotional resilience. By tending to your emotional health, you're better equipped to handle parenting's ups and downs with patience and empathy.

Examples: Practicing gratitude, giving yourself space to feel without judgment, and expressing emotions openly and honestly. This might also include setting aside time to process any frustrations or stress, whether through writing or talking with someone supportive, including a therapist.

Spiritual Self-Care

Spiritual self-care doesn't necessarily mean religious practice; it's about connecting with something greater, whether that's through nature, religion, meditation, or finding a sense of purpose. Spiritual self-care fosters a sense of peace and belonging, reminding you of your deeper values and helping you stay grounded.

Examples: Spending a few moments in meditation, visiting your place of worship, sitting quietly in nature, or reflecting on what brings meaning to your life. This can be as simple as setting aside time to connect with your inner self or finding activities that make you feel centered and whole.

Physical Self-Care

Physical self-care centers on taking care of your body's needs. A healthy body supports a healthy mind, giving you the stamina needed to handle daily challenges. Physical self-care can also relieve stress and provide a natural boost of energy, making it easier to approach parenting with patience and focus.

Examples: Taking a walk to get some fresh air, stretching, dancing, or engaging in any form of movement that feels good. This also includes ensuring you're getting enough sleep, staying hydrated, and nourishing your body with balanced meals.

Social Self-Care

Social self-care involves maintaining and nurturing relationships with those who support and energize you. While parenting can sometimes feel isolating, having a community you can rely on—friends, family, or even online parenting groups—can remind you that you're not alone. Social connections can help you recharge emotionally and provide a supportive outlet when things get tough.

Examples: Reaching out to a friend for a chat, planning a "date night" after the kids are in bed, joining a support group, or even scheduling regular check-ins with loved ones. Surrounding yourself with people who uplift you can make a big difference in your overall sense of well-being.

Intellectual Self-Care

Intellectual self-care is about challenging and expanding your mind. Engaging in learning and creative pursuits can give you a mental break from daily tasks, help you discover new interests, and boost your self-confidence. Intellectual stimulation helps keep your mind sharp and provides a sense of accomplishment and growth, which can energize you in other areas of life.

Examples: Reading a book, learning a new skill, solving puzzles, exploring a new hobby, or even listening to music that excites you. Intellectual self-care can be as simple as dedicating time each day to something that stimulates and interests you.

Each of these areas of self-care serves a different purpose, and you don't have to do them all to nurture yourself.

Choose two things that light you up and try them. Aim for one to two acts of self-care daily, even if each one lasts for only five minutes. Start small and build up.

And if you need to *trick* yourself into self-care to get started, know this: Self-care isn't just for you—it's a lesson for your child too. When your child sees you taking time for yourself, they learn the invaluable lesson that it's okay to take care of their own needs. They see that taking breaks, setting boundaries, and honoring personal well-being are important.

You're not just modeling how to be a parent—you're modeling how to be a whole person, one who knows how to find balance.

In the end, self-care is one of the greatest gifts you can give your child. Because when you're taken care of, you're able to show up as the calm, centered, and present parent they need.

Chapter 10
PARENTING TOGETHER

Parenting together isn't always the seamless partnership we imagine before kids enter the picture. Most of us don't sit down with our partners beforehand to have deep discussions about how we were raised, how we want to raise our kids, and how we'll handle specific behaviors and challenges. Instead, we dive in, muddling through babyhood in a fog of sleep deprivation and diaper changes, only to wake up one day with a limit-pushing toddler and parenting decisions that feel urgent, messy, and, sometimes, divided.

Conflict and disagreements are inevitable. But it's not because you're doing something wrong—it's because you and your partner are two unique individuals with your own histories, values, and perspectives. The fantasy of being perfectly aligned on every decision is just that: a fantasy. And holding on to that expectation often leads to frustration, miscommunication, and the very arguments we hoped to avoid.

The goal isn't to agree on everything but to find a way to work together. Parenting in harmony doesn't mean being on the same page all the time; it means being in the same book. It's about sharing a foundation of mutual goals for your child while respecting the different ways each of you might approach those goals. When you focus on your shared values and lean into each other's strengths, disagreements become opportunities to grow as a team—and as parents.

Same Book, Different Pages

It's morning, the clock is ticking, and your toddler has decided they *absolutely will not* put on clothes today. The goal is clear: You need to get out the door. But the bigger goal? Getting out the door *without* everyone yelling, crying, or storming off like they're actors in a soap opera. That's where teamwork comes in. You and your partner are in the same book—you both want a smooth and calm morning—but your pages might look different.

One parent might lean into choices: "Okay, do you want to get dressed now or after breakfast? It's up to you." This approach is about giving control and fostering independence. The toddler feels empowered, and the parent stays cool, calmly steering the situation.

The other parent might take the hands-on, playful route: "Hmm, are these clothes invisible? Or is your shirt hiding? Let's find it!" Suddenly, getting dressed turns into a game, complete with giggles and a race to see who can find the missing socks first.

Both approaches aim for the same thing: a dressed and reasonably happy child, and a morning that doesn't leave everyone frazzled. The magic? You're in sync on the *big goal*—but you don't have to tackle it the exact same way. Different strategies, same destination.

However, some parents might find themselves in completely different books, with one parent using a connection-based approach and the other using a compliance-at-all-costs approach. In that case, it's going to take more effort and a strong commitment to partnership to get into the same book.

Three Steps to Bridging the Gap in Differing Opinions

What happens when you and your partner aren't just in different books but seem to be in entirely different bookstores? That's when resentment and frustration can creep in, fueled by the temptation to focus on being right instead of working together.

The key? Shift the focus from being *right* to being *aligned*. The goal is to open the dialogue and find common ground without making anyone wrong. Here's how.

Step 1: Get Curious and Create a Connection

Start by seeking to understand, not to convince. Approach your partner's perspective with genuine curiosity.

- **Ask Thoughtful Questions:**
    - "How did it go for you when _____ happened?"
    - "What's your goal?"
    - "How does using this approach make you feel?"
    - "What impact does this approach have on our family?"

Then pause and listen.

When you listen without judgment or interjecting your own thoughts and emotions, you create a space where your partner feels safe to share. This reduces defensiveness and paves the way for productive conversation. Avoid slipping into attack mode—criticism only adds fuel to the fire. Instead, focus on connection, remembering that everyone is trying their best, even if their methods differ from yours. You might be surprised by what you discover when you take the time to truly listen.

Step 2: Talk About the Facts

Once you've listened and your partner feels heard, you can share your perspective—but with care.

- **Ask for Permission:** Before diving into your thoughts, invite the conversation:
    - "Can I share something with you?"
    - "Would it be okay if I told you about something I learned?"
- **Stick to the Facts:** Instead of focusing on opinions, share information:
    - "I read an article the other day that said . . ."
    - "I listened to a podcast that talked about this, and it was interesting . . ."

This shifts the conversation from "my way versus your way" to "something worth considering." It also takes the pressure off your partner to agree immediately, creating space for reflection. If your partner is more open, then you might try saying, "I've been trying ___ and here's what I noticed . . ."

Step 2.5: Get Curious Again

After sharing your perspective, turn the conversation back to your partner.

- **Ask Follow-Up Questions to Keep the Dialogue Open:**
    - "What do you think about this?"
    - "Have you ever heard about that before?"
    - "Would you be open to trying it?"

Humans are much more open to new ideas when they feel respected and included. If they sense they're being lectured or criticized, their walls will go up, and the conversation will stall. Re-centering the discussion around their thoughts encourages partnership and reduces resistance.

Step 3: Model the Behavior

Ultimately, you cannot control your parenting partner. The most powerful way to influence your co-parent is by modeling the behavior and approach you believe in.

- **Be the Change You Wish to See:** Demonstrate your philosophy through your actions. Let your partner see the positive results of your methods in real time. For example, if you want to focus on positive discipline, let your partner see it in action. If they notice your approach is defusing tantrums or creating connection, they'll likely grow curious: *What's working so well?*

When your co-parent notices progress—calmer transitions, fewer power struggles, or a more connected child—they may naturally wonder about what's working and want to join in. Focus on controlling what *you* can: your own thoughts, words, and actions.

PARENTING TOGETHER

> ### TODDLER TIP
> *What to Do When Your Parenting Partner*
> *Uses a Different Parenting Approach*
>
> There might still be moments when your partner parents differently than you would, perhaps leaning more into conventional approaches instead of what you believe is developmentally appropriate. That's okay. Your child will encounter plenty of people throughout their life—teachers, relatives, coaches—who don't handle things exactly the way you would. What matters most is how you help your child make sense of those experiences.
>
> If your partner's approach doesn't align with yours, focus on what *you* can control: how you respond and how you support your child. Validate their feelings—"How frustrating! You didn't like that Dad yelled at you"—and as they grow older, help them express those feelings directly to the other parent. This teaches your child not only emotional awareness but also how to navigate differences in relationships with confidence.

Being a Team, Even When You Disagree

Perhaps you set a limit around screen time, but your parenting partner tells your child it's okay to watch more. Frustrating? Absolutely. At its core, this kind of situation often comes down to differing views on how much screen time is acceptable—a challenge so many parents fail to agree on.

Here's the good news: You don't have to agree on everything to be a team.

Being a team doesn't mean you and your partner always see eye to eye or handle every situation the same way. What it *does* mean is that you find a way to show up together, even when you're not on the same page. It's about navigating those inevitable moments of disagreement without letting them derail your partnership—or confuse the heck out of your kid.

When your toddler's in the thick of it, the most important thing you can do is **show unity**. No, this doesn't mean you're silently endorsing what your partner just did. It means you're prioritizing consistency for your child in the moment and saving the "What the heck was that?" conversation for later. When one parent has started handling a situation, let them finish—even if you're dying to swoop in with your own approach. Unless someone's safety is at risk, stepping in only creates confusion and sets the stage for limit-pushing behavior.

Kids are *smart*. They'll sniff out even the tiniest crack in your parenting unity and start running through it. "Mom said no? Let's see what Dad says." This kind of limit-pushing behavior becomes more common as kids get older, but you have the chance to set the stage when they're young. Showing unity now teaches your child that the rules don't change depending on who they ask. This approach empowers both you and your parenting partner, reducing power struggles and preventing either of you from accidentally undermining the other.

TODDLER TIP
Get Ahead of a Situation

One way to make these moments smoother is by talking with your partner *before* these situations arise. Decide together how you'd like to handle disagreements in the moment. Create a plan for intervening—perhaps even come up with a simple phrase like "Do you need my help?" This allows the leading parent to either invite support or signal for space to handle things on their own. Having this agreement in place can prevent resentment and confusion and help you avoid stepping on each other's toes in the heat of the moment.

Now, here's where the real work happens: Once the dust settles, pull your co-parent aside (you know, when little ears aren't around) and have the conversation. No judgment, no accusations—just genuine curiosity. Maybe they didn't realize you'd already set a limit. Maybe they don't understand why you're so firm on this particular issue. Or maybe they just panicked and defaulted to what felt easiest in the moment. Whatever the case, start with "Hey, can we talk about what happened earlier?" and actually listen to what they have to say.

SCRIPTS FOR COMMUNICATION
Parenting Together

Your parenting partner just handled a challenging behavior situation with your child in a way you disagree with.

Avoid Shame and Anger
"Why did you say that? That is *not* the right way to respond."

Try Authentic Curiosity
"Can we recap what just happened? How was that for you? What do you feel worked? What do you feel didn't work?"

"I've noticed that trying _____ seems to help. Have you tried that before? What was your experience?"

Why It Works
Approaching with authentic curiosity opens up communication and minimizes defensiveness.

Always remember: The goal isn't perfect alignment; it's figuring out how to keep the big goal front of mind and how to respect each other's approaches enough to keep the wheels turning. Agree to back each other up in front of your child and keep working toward a longer-term plan.

Building teamwork as co-parents isn't a snap-your-fingers kind of deal. It's messy, it's a process, and it takes time. But even when you're not perfectly aligned, you can still raise your child as a united front. Being a team doesn't mean you have to agree on every little thing. It means you're committed to the big picture—raising a happy, well-adjusted kid who sees their parents working together, even when it's complicated.

Part 2

THE TODDLER EXPLAINED

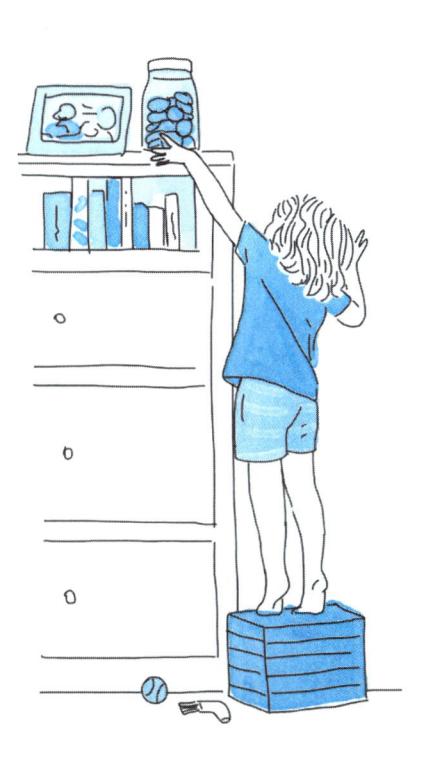

Chapter 11

UNDERSTANDING THE TODDLER BRAIN

Do you ever wonder what's happening inside of your toddler's head? One moment they're smiling and asking for a banana, and the next, they're freaking out as if the world has come crashing down because you dared to offer them that banana . . . *exactly as they requested*.

But fear not, because behind these confusing, contradictory, and (admittedly) frustrating shenanigans lies a fascinating realm of scientific discovery: the developing brain of a toddler. Over the past fifteen years, researchers and scientists have delved deeply into understanding the intricacies of toddler brain development, and what they've uncovered is not just a road map to navigating the tumultuous terrain of toddler behavior but also a profound insight into how these young minds perceive, learn, and interact with the world around them.

The Foundations of Toddler Brain Development

The toddler brain undergoes extraordinary growth in the early years until it is nearly full grown by age five. But what exactly is happening beneath the surface during this time?

From day one, your little love came equipped with about one hundred billion brain cells (or neurons)—roughly the same number as stars in the Milky Way. And as they grow, the number of connections, or synapses, between these neurons skyrockets. From birth to age five, a child's brain develops more rapidly than at any other time in life. During the first three years, your baby's brain is busy creating *more than a million* new neural connections every single second![1] When we talk about a brain being "wired," we're really talking about these synapses.

Quick Facts

- The brain doubles in size in a child's first year of life and keeps growing to about 80 percent of adult size by age three. By age five, a toddler's brain is nearly full grown at 90 percent.[2]
- The brain is built from the bottom up, starting before birth and continuing into adulthood (until about age twenty-five) when the brain is fully mature.[3]
- A newborn has all the neurons they'll have for the rest of their life, but what really makes the brain work are the connections (synapses).
- In the first few years of life, one million new neural pathways and connections form every second to build your child's brain architecture.[4]
- Simple connections and skills form first, then more complex circuits and skills.
- Circuits are connected through repeated use. The connections that are used become stronger and the ones that aren't used are pruned.
- The connections made in the first five years of life create either a firm or weak foundation for the connections that develop later.[5]

Because of all this, a child's experiences in the first five years have a profound impact on the rest of their lives. The more a pathway is used, the stronger it becomes. For example, if a child is exposed to spanking, constant yelling, or other fear-based parenting approaches, the pathways for the fear response will become stronger.

Additionally, if your toddler is frequently exposed to yelling, they may learn to express frustration in similar ways. If they encounter withdrawal, stonewalling, or silence, their brain may learn to mirror these behaviors in their own interactions. This reflection goes beyond simple mimicry—it's powered by **mirror neurons**, specialized cells in the brain that allow your child to internalize and replicate what they observe.

Mirror neurons play a critical role in learning and emotional development, helping toddlers understand and imitate the behaviors, emotions, and intentions of those around them. When you model calm responses, empathy, and problem-solving, you're essentially "programming" their brain to mirror those positive behaviors. Conversely, if they're exposed to repeated negative patterns, their mirror neurons will pick up on and embed those habits as well.

The Downstairs and Upstairs Brain

As with any architectural masterpiece, the stability of the brain's final structure depends on the integrity of its foundation. According to the Center on the Developing Child at Harvard University, it is easiest to form strong brain circuits during the early years when the brain's plasticity is at its highest; the older we get, the more physiologically costly intervention becomes.[6] Brains, again, are built over time, layer by layer, from the ground up. In *The Whole-Brain Child* by Daniel J. Siegel and Tina Payne Bryson, the "upstairs brain" and "downstairs brain" are metaphors used to describe the two main areas of the brain and how they influence behavior, especially in children.[7]

The Downstairs Brain: Brain Stem and Limbic Region

The "downstairs brain" refers to the more primitive parts of your toddler's brain, which develop first.

The downstairs brain is responsible for
- basic functions (breathing, blinking, and swallowing),

- innate reactions, impulses, and stress responses (fight, flight, freeze, fawn), and
- emotions (including anger and fear).[8]

Your toddler spends a lot of time in this area of the brain. This explains why toddlers can exhibit intense emotional outbursts or impulsive actions seemingly without forethought.

The Upstairs Brain: Cerebral Cortex

This is the more evolved, sophisticated part of your child's brain, which includes the prefrontal cortex.

The upstairs brain is responsible for

- complex mental processes,
- analytical thinking and planning (considering consequences to actions),
- impulse control (thinking before acting),
- problem-solving and logical thinking (including decision-making skills),
- emotional regulation (leading to behavioral regulation), and
- empathy (considering how others feel).[9]

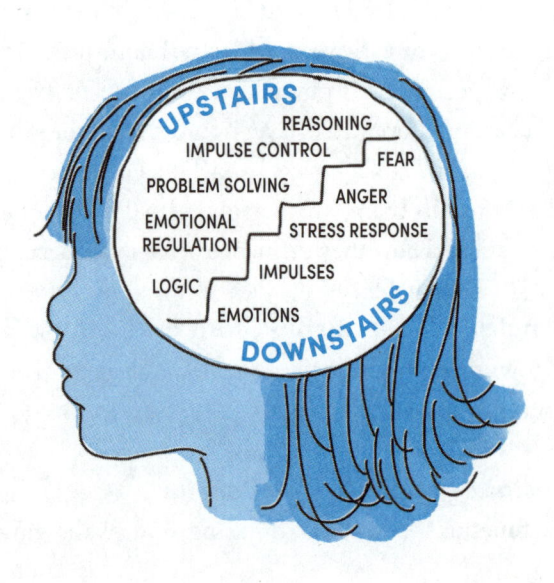

This is the last area of the brain to develop and only begins to mature at a more rapid pace around the age of four.

In a nutshell? The downstairs brain is the emotional epicenter, the part of the brain responsible for our immediate reactions and survival instincts. The upstairs brain is the sophisticated control center, responsible for executive functions such as decision-making, problem-solving, and emotional regulation. So when your toddler is overwhelmed or stressed, it's the *downstairs* brain that's in overdrive. They might be melting down over a spilled cup of milk, a broken toy, or getting that banana they asked for—whatever their reaction, it's merely an indicator that their emotions are swirling uncontrollably. In other words: *It's not their fault!* What's more, using fear as a parenting tool keeps children in their downstairs brain.

Kids need to be in their upstairs brain to learn skills and be in control of their behavior. It's our job to walk them from their lower brain back to their upper brain. We do this by helping a child feel seen, heard, safe, and loved, which can be achieved through some of the following strategies:

- **Responsive Parenting:** By responding consistently and empathetically to a toddler's emotional needs and behaviors, parents help strengthen neural connections associated with emotional regulation through coregulation.
- **Creating Secure Attachment:** One of the most critical pieces of a baby and toddler's life is to have a secure attachment with at least one adult. Toddlers need a parent or primary caregiver who offers them a sense of safety no matter what they do or how they act in any given moment, who comforts them when they're experiencing big emotions that they don't know how to control, and who acknowledges that their feelings are valid.
- **Eliminating Toxic Stress:** Not all stress is harmful. **Positive stress** creates resilience by teaching children how to adapt and cope with challenges, especially when buffered by loving, supportive relationships. For example, brief stress, like adjusting to a new caregiver or falling down, helps build healthy stress-response systems when these stressors are met with support from a trusted adult.

However, **toxic stress** harms brain development when a child faces prolonged, unbuffered adversity—such as abuse, neglect, or chronic exposure to stressful situations (e.g., spanking and constant yelling). This kind of stress can negatively impact the brain's architecture and stress-response systems, with lifelong effects on learning and behavior, as well as physical and emotional health. Parents can mitigate toxic stress by providing a safe, nurturing environment and fostering strong, supportive relationships that protect a child's developing brain.[10]

> **Positive stress** = a challenging situation in which we have a sense of control or feel supported in navigating
>
> **Toxic stress** = a threatening situation that goes on and on, and that we don't feel capable of getting through

Consistent positive interactions create a nurturing environment that supports healthy brain development. When toddlers feel safe, loved, and understood, they are more likely to thrive emotionally, socially, and intellectually.

I want to be clear: This doesn't mean parents need to be perfect—far from it! You're human, and mistakes are inevitable. But the good news is that mistakes are learning opportunities in disguise. Instead of striving for perfection, focus on repairing and reconnecting when things go sideways. When you model repairing a relationship, you're teaching your child how to do the same. They're learning from you that it's okay to mess up and that relationships can be strengthened through repair.

What truly matters is the quality and consistency of your responses. Remember, consistency doesn't mean getting it right 100 percent of the time—it means that, more often than not, your child can count on you to respond in a predictable and reassuring way. This sense of predictability provides the security toddlers need as they navigate their world.

Remember, practice makes progress, not perfection.

And here's the best part: Because this time of brain development is so rapid, it means *nothing is permanent.* That period of them waking up five times a night leaving you exhausted and depleted? That's a common phase linked to sleep regressions due to those rapid changes in their brain. The biting, temper tantrums, and phases of clinginess? They will pass. These moments are simply part of the larger tapestry of growth, a testament to the whirlwind of development that is happening inside your child's brain.

My invitation to you is to embrace these times with patience and understanding, knowing that they are just chapters in a much larger story. (No matter how bananas they may feel.)

Chapter 12

GETTING TO KNOW YOUR TODDLER'S SENSORY SYSTEM

It's a sunny Saturday, and you and your little one are in the car heading to the park. Suddenly your toddler starts kicking and screaming. Thoughts race through your head: *Why is he crying?! Is this because I said no to the ice cream ten minutes ago? Is he hungry? Tired? Does he hate Taylor Swift? (Impossible.)*

As a parent, it can be challenging to discover and respond to a child's behavior and needs—especially when you don't know what they are! To truly understand what's driving your child's behavior, it's vital to view these situations through not only a behavioral lens but also a *sensory* lens.

The sensory system helps us process the world and makes us aware of how we feel in our own bodies. We all know the five main senses: sight, smell, taste, hearing, and touch. But did you know there are actually *eight* senses total? These are the three additional senses:

1. **Vestibular Sense:** Located in the inner ear, this sense helps us understand the body's position relative to gravity and space. It informs our sense of balance, movement, and spatial awareness, contributing to motor skills and overall alertness. Anytime we

make a change in our head position, the fluid in our inner ears lets us know where we are (which is how we get that feeling of dizziness or motion sickness). This sense is active even before birth, as we move within the womb.

2. **Interoceptive Sense:** This sense relates to internal sensations from our organs, such as hunger, temperature, thirst, and heart rate. It is crucial for emotional regulation and mindfulness, helping us understand and respond to our internal states.
3. **Proprioceptive Sense:** This is your body's internal navigation system letting you know the position and movement of your body parts in relation to each other and your environment. It detects how your muscles, tendons, and joints are moving and stretching, allowing you to perform tasks like walking in the dark or dressing without needing to see yourself. (For instance, you never really have to *think* about putting your arms through the sleeves of your shirt . . . at least most of the time.)

In every moment our brains collect information from our senses that tells us about the world around us. **Sensory processing** is the brain's way of organizing and interpreting sensory information automatically and unconsciously from all eight senses. **Sensory modulation** is how the brain prioritizes this information and responds to it. For many of us, this happens effortlessly, allowing us to regulate our responses to various stimuli. However, for young children, especially toddlers, this system is still developing and can be easily overwhelmed, dysregulated, or even understimulated. For example, some kids might over-respond to loud noises and cover their ears, while other children might under-respond and not be aware of their surroundings.

That minivan meltdown could have been caused by any number of reasons that your child may not have been able to pinpoint: Maybe the AC was too low, the seat belt was digging into their arm, or—and I hesitate to say it!—they have the audacity not to love Taylor Swift. (It's okay, they'll learn in time.)

Whatever the reason, it's important to know that daily sensory stimuli have an impact on your child's behavior.

Supporting Sensory Regulation

When a child's sensory system is out of balance, they may seek more or less input to regulate themself. Some children seek out sensory experiences—craving deep-pressure hugs, spinning, or jumping—charging through their day with unstoppable energy. Others may be highly sensitive to sensory stimuli, hitting the brakes and withdrawing from the chaos in search of calm when faced with loud noises, scratchy clothing, or crowded spaces. Understanding these behaviors isn't about fixing them—it's about recognizing how our children's bodies are trying to find balance and helping them get there.

Sensory Seekers: Craving More Input

Picture a toddler on a mission: jumping, climbing, crashing—relentless in their pursuit of adventure. Does this sound familiar? Then that means you have a little sensory seeker! These sensory seekers aren't being wild for the sake of it; they're responding to a deep, internal need for stimulation. Every touch, sound, and movement helps them feel more connected to the world. Supporting them means creating opportunities to move and get enough sensory input to regulate themselves.

Common Sensory-Seeking Behaviors and Potential Signs Your Child Needs More Sensory Input

- exhibiting restlessness or having trouble sitting still
- constantly moving, climbing, or jumping
- frequently crashing into objects or people
- speaking fast or overly loud
- having low body awareness
- pushing feet into things
- touching everything, often seeming impulsive
- making loud noises or enjoying noisy environments
- chewing on objects like clothing or toys

How to Support Sensory Seekers

- **Create Opportunities for Movement:** Offer activities like trampoline

jumping, swinging, marching, crawling, and setting up simple obstacle courses to get their body moving.
- **Provide Fidget Tools:** Use items like stress balls, fidget spinners, or chewy necklaces for oral sensory input.
- **Incorporate Heavy Work Activities:** Encourage tasks like carrying groceries, pushing a full laundry basket, or doing wall pushes.
- **Schedule Regular Sensory Breaks:** Build active breaks into daily routines to help maintain focus and calm.
- **Provide Deep Pressure:** Wind down with calming activities such as lightly squishing them, giving compression hugs, using a weighted blanket, or having your child squeeze a body pillow to promote relaxation.

Sensory Avoiders: Needing Less Input

Now think of a toddler who seems to shrink back when the world feels too loud, too bright, or too unpredictable. These sensory avoiders aren't shy—they're protective. Their finely tuned senses can get overwhelmed by what seems ordinary to others. They're not being difficult when they resist new textures or noisy spaces—they're seeking refuge from a world that sometimes feels like too much. Supporting them means creating safe, predictable spaces where they can breathe easier and explore at their own pace.

Common Sensory-Avoiding Behaviors and Potential Signs Your Child Needs Less Sensory Input

- covering ears or eyes frequently
- avoiding certain foods due to texture
- becoming overwhelmed by loud or chaotic environments
- avoiding messy play like finger painting or sandboxes
- being hypersensitive to clothing textures, tags, or certain fabrics
- startling easily at sudden noises or touches

How to Support Sensory Avoiders

- **Create a Calm-Down Space:** Set up a quiet, cozy corner with dim lighting and soft blankets.

- **Use Noise-Canceling Earmuffs/Headphones:** Help reduce overwhelming auditory input in noisy settings. Hang them on a low hook so your child can access them as needed.
- **Offer Predictable Routines:** Consistency can reduce sensory-related anxiety.
- **Introduce New Sensory Experiences Gradually:** Allow exploration at the child's pace to build tolerance.

For sensory avoiders who are still learning to manage sensory processing, their brains might interpret a loud noise or a glaring light as overwhelming. In that moment they become dysregulated, and their immediate reaction could be covering their ears or eyes, or even more intense behaviors like crying or fleeing. This is just the brain's way of managing sensory overload.

Conversely, for sensory seekers who crave movement and feel confined during circle time, their brain might urge them to jump or move around—so crisscross applesauce isn't going to cut it. It might seem like they're not paying attention or they're disregarding safety, but in reality, their brains are signaling a need for more sensory stimulation in order to stay engaged and focused. The brain says, "Ya gotta get up and jump!" So they will get up and jump.

Understanding these connections helps us see that behavior is often just a reflection of how a child is processing and responding to sensory information. So often we assume a toddler is being disrespectful or rude when, in actuality, that toddler is just trying to meet a need and communicate something.

Making Sense of the World

Just as adults have preferences for certain environments or sensations, children, too, exhibit unique sensory preferences. Understanding your child's sensory preferences can help you understand their behavior and more effectively respond to and prevent challenging behaviors.

Start by observing patterns and writing down what you notice. Pay attention to what seems to help them feel calm and regulated—like a tight hug, a massage, or a sip of water. Notice what their body needs more of and what they seem to avoid. Many toddlers show mixed sensory preferences—seeking input in one area (like movement) while avoiding it in another (like loud noises).

Identify any recurring patterns. For instance, is it a particular sound, a type of fabric, or a lack of movement that affects them? By organizing this information, you can gain a clearer sense of what your child needs when they don't have the words to express it, and you can learn how to better adapt to their needs. For example, this might involve providing gloves for sensory play.

By having a deeper understanding of their unique sensory system, you can provide your kiddo with tailor-made ways to regulate themselves and make appropriate choices when dysregulation strikes. Focus on being curious and observant, and then build from there.

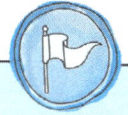

RED FLAG
Sensory Processing Challenges

Some children are more acutely impacted by their environment and experience emotions more deeply. If your toddler covers their ears when hearing loud noises, complains about tags in their clothing, or has an extra-difficult time with transitions but can adapt with support, they may have sensory processing sensitivity (SPS), also known as being a highly sensitive person (HSP). This is a natural personality trait that is present in 10 to 20 percent of the population. People with this trait have heightened sensitivity to lights, sound, touch, and tastes, resulting in resisting certain clothing and food textures; being overwhelmed by loud sounds, strong smells, and bright lights; and experiencing heightened emotional reactivity.

In contrast, sensory processing disorder (SPD) is a neurological condition that involves significant challenges in processing and responding to sensory information, causing over-responsiveness and under-responsiveness to sensory stimuli that leads to severe meltdowns and interferes with daily activities. It sometimes exists alongside other neurodevelopmental conditions, such as autism spectrum disorder (ASD) and attention deficit hyperactivity disorder (ADHD). If you are concerned about your child's development, sensory system, or behavior, consider consulting a developmental pediatrician or pediatric occupational therapist for evaluation and guidance. Early understanding leads to better support!

Bottom line: If your child's behavior is so intense that it's disrupting the entire family and derailing you from being able to do day-to-day activities, it's best to consult your pediatrician to refer you to the appropriate specialists based on your child's specific needs.

Chapter 13

SETTING REALISTIC EXPECTATIONS

Here's the deal: It's not that your toddler won't do what you're asking. It's that they *can't*. Your child's inability to behave is about their lack of skills and brain maturation, not their desire.

As parents, we often fall into the trap of expecting our children to behave in a way that, developmentally, they aren't yet capable of. According to one early childhood organization's National Parent Survey, "About half of parents believe that children are capable of self-control and other developmental milestones much earlier than they actually are."[1] This expectation gap is at the heart of much of the frustration and tension we experience as parents and caregivers. But what if we could shift our perspective and align our expectations with the realities of toddler development? What if we could meet our children where they are instead of where we think they should be? When we are able to do this, parenting becomes a lot easier and a lot less frustrating.

The Reality of Toddler Development

These are some of the common misconceptions about toddler capabilities, according to recent surveys:

- A little less than half (43 percent) of parents thought children younger than age two can share and take turns with their peers. And more than 71 percent believed children have this ability by the time they are three. In reality, this skill typically develops between ages three and four.
- About a third (36 percent) of parents believed children under age two can resist the desire to do something forbidden, and more than half (56 percent) said this level of impulse control is gained before age three. In truth, most children don't begin to master this until they are between three and a half to four years of age, and full mastery can take several more years.[2]

These statistics reveal a significant gap between what we expect our children to do and what they are capable of doing. It's no wonder so many parents (and toddlers!) feel frustrated and overwhelmed!

The Impact of Misaligned Expectations

When we expect our toddlers to behave in ways that are beyond their developmental capabilities, we set ourselves up for disappointment and set them up for failure.

The thing is, we often underestimate a toddler's physical abilities and overestimate their emotional-regulation abilities. Here are two relatable examples:

- **Your Toddler Can:** put on their shoes or feed themselves, but you might do these things for them because it's faster or you are afraid they might get hurt.
- **But They Can't:** stop a tantrum when they feel emotionally or sensorily overwhelmed. Their brains aren't developed enough to manage that level of emotional control.

This mismatch between expectations and your child's developmental reality can lead to a cycle of negative interactions. You expect more than your toddler can give, they don't meet those expectations, you get frustrated, and they respond to your frustration with more challenging behavior.

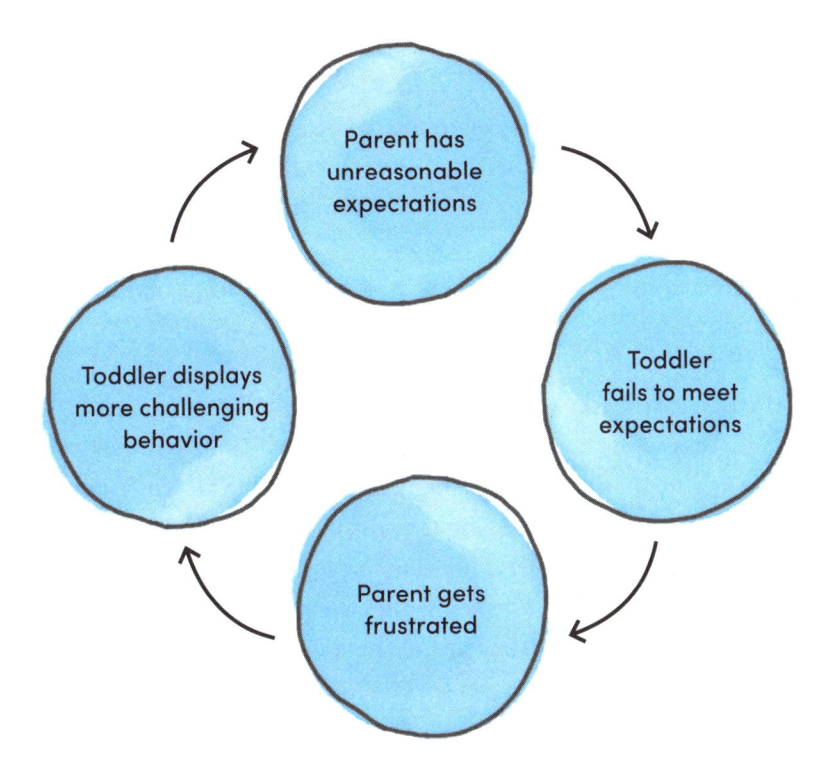

```
         Parent has
        unreasonable
         expectations
    ↗                    ↘
Toddler displays         Toddler
more challenging      fails to meet
   behavior            expectations
    ↖                    ↙
         Parent gets
          frustrated
```

This is why it's important to remember your toddler's meltdown or refusal to comply isn't defiance; it's *communication*. They're telling you, "This is too much for me right now!" or "I need to feel more in control." It bears repeating: *Your child's inability to behave is about their lack of skill and brain maturation, not their desire.* Many times your toddler is not developmentally able to meet your expectations. A toddler can only do what their brain is capable of doing!

Toddlers Are Not Yet Capable Of

- **Understanding Time:** Abstract concepts like "five more minutes" are beyond their grasp.
- **Controlling Their Emotions When Upset:** Their brains are still developing the ability to manage big feelings.

- **Considering the Feelings of Others:** Empathy is a skill that emerges gradually with brain maturation and modeling.
- **Thinking Rationally and Logically:** They are driven by emotion and impulse, not logic.
- **Expressing Their Emotions with Words:** Limited vocabulary makes it hard for them to communicate complex feelings.
- **Sharing Their Toys with Others:** Toddlerhood is an egocentric period of development where children think everything is because of them or for them.
- **Consistently Controlling Their Impulses:** Acting on immediate desires is developmentally appropriate for this age.

Picture this: You tell your two-year-old, "We're leaving in five minutes," expecting them to start wrapping up their play. But when the time comes to go, they dissolve into a full-blown meltdown. You might feel angry or frustrated, thinking they're being stubborn or defiant. But the reality is, toddlers don't understand abstract concepts like time yet. They're not resisting on purpose—they simply can't grasp what "five minutes" means or what's expected of them in that context.

Meeting Your Child Where They Are

So what's the solution? It starts with a shift in mindset. Instead of asking, *How do I make my child listen?* start asking yourself if your expectations are realistic given their developmental stage. This isn't about lowering standards; it's about aligning them with what's actually possible for your child at this moment in their development. Then ask yourself, *What skills does my child need to learn to be successful here?* Instead of focusing on what your toddler *can't* do, celebrate what they *can* do, and gently guide them toward the next step in their development.

Four Practical Strategies for Setting Realistic Expectations

1. **Educate Yourself:** Understanding the typical milestones for toddler development can help you set more realistic expectations.

When you know what's typical, you're less likely to set unrealistic standards and be frustrated when your child doesn't meet them.

2. **Get Curious:** When you find yourself frustrated with your child's behavior, take a moment to ask, *Is this something they're capable of right now?* If the answer is no, adjust your expectations accordingly.

3. **Use Scaffolding:** Scaffolding is like giving your toddler a boost to reach the next step. It's a teaching strategy that is all about offering *just enough* support to help them succeed—lining up their shoes so they can put them on or steadying them on a step before letting go. As they gain confidence, you gradually step back and let them take the lead. It's not about doing it for them; it's about guiding them until they're ready to soar on their own.

4. **Provide Support and Guidance:** Rather than expecting your child to figure things out on their own, offer support and guidance. Help them navigate their emotions, understand social rules, and practice self-control in a way that's appropriate for their developmental stage.

Understanding that toddlers are not miniature adults is critical. Their developmental drive to experiment and explore is stronger than their brain maturation and life experience, often leading to impulsive behaviors that challenge our patience but are completely normal for their stage of growth. They aren't being difficult on purpose; they're exploring their world the only way they know how.

Developing Impulse Control

Everything in the checkout line is new, shiny, and perfectly positioned at their eye level. It's a sensory wonderland begging to be touched. Your toddler is captivated, reaching for items faster than you can redirect them. Sound familiar?

While this might feel like a test of your patience, moments like these are opportunities to connect and teach. Instead of jumping to frustration, try acknowledging their curiosity and struggle.

For example, you might say, "You really want to grab that toy, and you're having a hard time stopping yourself." Then offer an alternative: "Look with your eyes, please. What do you see?"

If the reaching continues, follow through calmly: "You're still trying to touch it. I'm going to help you stop by moving you back."

Supporting your toddler doesn't mean yelling, threatening, or punishing—it means setting limits and helping them meet those limits in a way that fosters learning. You can also redirect their curiosity by letting them explore safe items, like the ones already in your cart.

And remember, this process takes time. Impulse control doesn't develop overnight. Your little one has only been on this earth for one to four years, while you've had decades to practice self-control. The journey may be messy, but with realistic expectations and consistent guidance, you can support your toddler as they grow into their potential.

Many parents ask me, "How can you tell if your expectations are too high for your toddler?" My answer: *Their behavior will show you.* If they consistently struggle to meet what you're asking, it's a sign they aren't yet developmentally ready. But this doesn't mean you should simply wait for them to grow out of it. You have the ability to influence their development and help them build the skills they need to succeed.

Impulse control isn't something toddlers are born with—it's a skill they learn over time through practice. Since the prefrontal cortex is still developing, toddlers are naturally impulsive. But with your guidance, they can build self-regulation through fun, interactive strategies. Games that involve stopping, waiting, and following directions are excellent tools for teaching impulse control. Try these classics:

- **Red Light, Green Light:** Practice stopping and starting on command.
- **Simon Says:** Teach listening skills and the ability to pause before acting.
- **Freeze Tag:** Encourage quick thinking and stopping when tagged.
- **Musical Chairs:** Practice moving with intention and stopping suddenly.

When we align our expectations with our children's *actual* developmental abilities, we create an environment where everyone can thrive. We move from a place of constant correction and frustration to one of support and encouragement (and real joy!). By recognizing where our children are in their journey, we not only reduce the stress in our lives but also empower our toddlers to grow into confident, capable individuals.

Bridging the expectation gap isn't about lowering standards or giving in to every whim. It's about meeting your child where they are, celebrating their progress, and guiding them toward their next developmental milestones with love and understanding.

Chapter 14

DECODING TODDLER BEHAVIOR

Your toddler is not bad, rude, mean, or manipulative. Sure, it can feel that way when they're lying on the floor in the middle of Target, wailing because you wouldn't buy them a new dinosaur. But what if I told you that meltdown isn't a sign of moral failure (on their part or yours)? It's just the most effective way your toddler knows to get their needs met in that moment.

So let's start by clearing up the common misconception that toddlers are manipulative. The truth is: *Toddlers are strategic, not manipulative.* There's a big difference. Manipulation implies scheming—an intentional attempt to deceive. Toddlers don't have the developmental chops for that kind of emotional chess game. They are tiny scientists, experimenting with trial and error to figure out what works to get their needs and desires met. Most of your child's behavior is trying to get their physical, emotional, and developmental needs met.

If whining gets them the fruit snack, they'll log that as a success. If a tantrum in the store scores them a new toy, you better believe they'll try it again. This is strategic. It doesn't mean you're a bad parent, and it doesn't make them a bad kid. It's simply how they're wired to communicate.

Behavior Is Not Good or Bad

When we interpret a child's behavior as disrespectful or bratty, it pulls us into defensive mode. Suddenly, we're feeling disrespected, frustrated, and gearing up for battle. But what if we took a step back? What if we saw their behavior not as a challenge to our authority but as a message? Instead of shutting down the behavior with punishment, try getting curious to understand what's beneath it.

So often we label our toddlers' behavior as good or bad, but behavior is neutral! It's simply how our bodies act and move in an environment. Sure, hitting and pushing are behaviors (and understandably behaviors you want to see less of!), but coughing and lifting your knee are behaviors as well. When we focus solely on stopping the behavior—making the screaming, hitting, or whining go away—we reduce the child to being "bad," "rude," or even "manipulative." But when we shift our perspective and approach behavior as a form of communication, we open the door to curiosity and connection. And it's in that connection where true transformation happens—for both your response and your toddler's behavior.

At their core, labels are judgments—interpretations of what's happening and not actual facts. Labels help us make sense of the chaos, categorizing feelings, experiences, environments, and even people, but labeling behavior as "good" or "bad" is also the number one obstacle to decoding toddler behavior and parenting your child in a developmentally appropriate way. And here's the kicker: Those labels, whether intended or not, can *stick*.

Over time, labels have the following consequences:

- **Labels Shape Identity:** A child labeled as "bad" may internalize that label, and this may reinforce challenging behavior.
- **Labels Affect How You Treat Them:** A "troublemaker" may find it harder to receive empathy from their caregiver, even in moments when they're genuinely trying to do better.
- **Labels Limit Potential:** Even positive labels, like "smart" or "kind," can box a child into specific roles, creating pressure to always perform or behave a certain way.

When we label a toddler's behavior as "good," "bad," "naughty," or "rude," we place a heavy weight on tiny shoulders. Labels like "good" or "bad" are judgments that reflect our own interpretations, not what's truly happening. Looking at behavior through this lens disempowers us and makes parenting harder.

Consequences of Focusing Solely on Correcting "Bad" or Eliciting "Good" Behavior

- You're more likely to feel triggered, frustrated, and compelled to control your toddler's actions.
- Curiosity takes a back seat, making it harder to understand what's driving the behavior.
- The emphasis shifts to punishment as a quick fix to stop the behavior, which can unintentionally shut down your toddler's emotions and block true learning and behavior transformation.
- Toddlers end up being punished for expressing their needs and feelings in ways that reflect their still-developing brain and limited life experience.

Let's face it: Dropping the habit of labeling isn't easy because it's usually deeply ingrained in us. But with practice, it can transform the way you see and respond to your child.

TODDLER TIP
Observe and Describe Behavior

Instead of making judgments, try observing and describing the behavior. The goal is to stay neutral and repeat the facts.

For example, instead of saying, "That was mean," try, "You hit me when I said no."

This approach focuses on the action rather than assigning

> blame or a moral judgment, making it easier to understand and address the root cause. Our focus moves from simply stopping the behavior to understanding what's behind it—whether it's feelings, emotions, unmet needs, or developmental stages. When we shift from viewing behavior through a labeling lens to seeing all behavior as communication, something transformative happens.

Toddler Behavior: The Tip of the Iceberg

When you shift from labeling to observing and describing, you start to see your child's behavior in a new light, allowing you the space to uncover what they're really communicating.

Toddlers rarely say "I'm having a tough day" with words—they show us with their behavior.

At first glance, you may see behaviors like these that, on the surface, seem loud, messy, and completely overwhelming:

- screaming
- hitting
- throwing
- whining

But that's just the tip of the iceberg. Beneath the surface lies a wealth of feelings, emotions, unmet needs, and desires that your toddler doesn't yet have the tools to articulate.

Here's what might really be going on:

- "I'm hungry or tired."
- "I need to feel loved and connected."
- "I'm struggling to cope with being told no."
- "I'm overwhelmed and need a break."
- "I'm feeling powerless."

The behavior we see on the surface is not the whole story of your child's behavior. In fact, it's a very small part. To truly understand and transform behavior, you have to uncover and address the root.

The Root of Behavior

Your toddler doesn't wake up thinking, *How can I make my parent's life miserable today?* Their outbursts, refusals, and tears are a normal part of being a toddler—how you interpret and respond to their behavior is what creates effective parenting. It starts with this perspective shift.

> All behavior is communication. It's not "bad." It's your toddler's way of asking for help in getting their needs met.

This perspective shift—seeing behavior as communication instead of defiance—doesn't just help you respond more calmly. It strengthens your relationship with your child, creating a foundation of trust and connection that will last well beyond the toddler years.

Results of Approaching Behavior as Communication
- We open the door to connection, compassion, and empathy. Instead of thinking, *My toddler is being bad,* we recognize, *My toddler is having a hard time and needs my support.*
- Our stress response softens. We're less likely to react emotionally because we're approaching the situation with curiosity rather than judgment.

Imagine: You're sick, tired, hungry, frustrated, alone, or scared—and no one is helping you. You try to explain how you feel, but your words aren't coming out right, or worse, no one is listening. How would you respond? Chances are, you'd do what it takes to be seen and heard.

That's what's happening with your toddler. *They're not giving you a hard time; they're* having *a hard time.* With that understanding, you're no longer battling against them and their behavior—you're partnering with them to uncover what they truly need.

No matter how frustratingly cryptic it seems, your toddler's behavior is communicating these four things:

1. **Feelings and Emotions:** These are expressed physically during the toddler years. Toddlers may not have the words to articulate their feelings, so they use actions.
2. **Needs:** Behaviors can signal **basic needs** like hunger and tiredness; the need to be heard; the need for connection and feeling unconditionally loved; and the need to feel safe. They also communicate **developmental needs** like the need to experiment, explore, and move; the need to feel capable and independent; and the need to belong and have a sense of control or power. **Sensory needs** also play a role—some toddlers seek more input (movement, noise, touch), while others avoid it (bright lights, strong smells, crowds).
3. **Brain Maturation:** With developing impulse control and emotional regulation, toddlers struggle to calm themselves and need help co-regulating. Their behavior reflects their brain's growth, not defiance.
4. **Temperament:** Every child has a unique temperament that shapes how they react, regulate emotions, and adapt to new experiences. Some are flexible, others need routine. Recognizing their reactivity, self-regulation, and sociability helps in responding with patience and support.

It's okay if you don't always know the *exact* need driving your toddler's behavior. Sometimes the tantrum is a clear signal—hunger, tiredness, frustration—and sometimes it's a mystery wrapped in an enigma. You're not failing as a parent when you can't figure it out. The real power lies in simply knowing that *there's always something underneath the behavior.*

Remember: Your toddler is so much more than their behavior. You are so much more than your reactions to your toddler's behavior. You and your toddler are human and are learning along the way.

TODDLER BEHAVIOR DECODER

Understanding your toddler's behavior starts with recognizing that what you see on the surface isn't the whole story—it's their way of communicating big feelings and unmet needs in the only ways they know how.

Toddler Appears	*Toddler Actually Is*
defiant	practicing autonomy
manipulative	strategic in meeting a need or desire
bad	struggling to cope
needy	looking for connection
difficult	having a hard time

Behavior on the Surface	*What It Really Means*
"No!"	They are exerting independence and learning they can set boundaries.
tantruming	They are experiencing sensory/emotional overwhelm and are unable to cope—an emotional "poop" or release of pent-up feelings.
"I don't like you" or "You're mean"	They are struggling to accept a limit or expressing frustration with not liking what you're saying.
avoiding eye contact after breaking rules	They are feeling embarrassed or ashamed because they couldn't resist their impulses.
laughing when you lose patience	They are feeling uncomfortable or nervous and are reacting to intense emotions they don't know how to handle.

Chapter 15

REDEFINING DISCIPLINE

Discipline is so much more than setting limits and trying to make your child listen to you; it's about teaching. But for too long, discipline has been a stand-in for punishment. The go-to tools—threats or bribes, ignoring children or issuing time-outs, spanking and yelling—are all rooted in a deep-seated desire to control the child and make them obey. We knowingly and sometimes unknowingly resort to blame, shame, guilt, judgment, or outright overpowering a child to instill fear and enforce obedience. The goal? Compliance at any cost. The result? A child who may follow directions out of fear—not understanding—and a dynamic where short-term obedience is achieved at the expense of emotional growth, self-regulation, and long-term connection.

Here's how **conventional discipline** tends to play out:

You're making dinner, barely holding it together, when—*crash*. Juice everywhere. The cup you just told your kid not to mess with is now shattered on the floor.

Frustration takes over. "I told you not to do that! Go to your room!"

Your edict is met with tears. Stomping. A slammed door. And for a moment, there's silence.

But what did they *actually* learn? Probably not what you hoped. More likely, they learned that mistakes equal punishment, that big feelings should be handled alone, and that you're the enemy when they mess up.

Now, if you're reading this and thinking, *OMG, I've been doing it all wrong*, stop. Breathe. You are not bad or wrong—you are human. This is an invitation to pivot, learn, and embrace a more effective way.

If you're thinking, *I'm the adult, and my child needs to listen and respect me when I ask them to do something*, well then, let's pause for a moment. Ask yourself: *What's the real goal here?* Is it just compliance, or is it something deeper?

Discipline that focuses solely on obedience is shortsighted. Sure, you might get your child to do what you want in the moment, but it comes at a cost. It doesn't address the root cause of their behavior, and it misses an opportunity to teach the skills they need to manage themself in the future when you aren't around. Instead, it often punishes a child for being exactly what they are—human, imperfect, and learning. To raise an emotionally healthy, confident child, we need to focus on teaching kids skills, *not* punishing them for a lack of skills.

TODDLER TIP
Why Spanking Isn't the Answer

Spanking might stop a behavior in the moment, but at what cost? Over fifty years of research shows that spanking doesn't teach—it harms. It increases aggression, lowers self-esteem, and damages the parent-child relationship.[1] Toddlers don't stop because they've learned a better way; they stop because they're afraid of losing your love and acceptance—two things they need to thrive.

Put Yourself in Their Shoes

Now, picture this: You're at work, juggling a million things, and your boss comes over, barking orders. You hesitate for a moment, maybe because you're overwhelmed, confused, or need clarification. Instead of addressing the situation with understanding, your boss yells at you, threatens to dock your pay, or sends you to the corner to "think about your actions." How do you feel? Respected? Motivated to try harder? Or resentful, embarrassed, and less inclined to give your best effort?

Or consider your spouse. Let's say you forget to take out the trash because you're exhausted from a long day. Instead of recognizing your fatigue or asking why it wasn't done, they give you the cold shoulder, snap at you, or declare, "No Netflix tonight since you can't follow through." Does this inspire love and cooperation—or frustration and disconnection?

When fear, shame, or control become our go-to discipline tools, the unintended message we send to our kids is clear: "You're bad for making a mistake." Because toddlerhood is an egocentric developmental period, instead of understanding why their behavior was an issue or learning how to make better choices, they either comply out of fear or dig in and push back even harder. Focusing on control and compliance often leads to frustration for everyone. In contrast, effective discipline focuses on skill building, allowing you to meet your toddler where they are, build a connection, and guide them toward learning the skills they need to develop impulse control.

So the next time you're in that moment, ask yourself: *What is my goal? Is it short-term compliance or long-term growth?* Instead of asking, *What punishment or consequence does my child need for this behavior?* try asking, *What skill does my child need to learn to navigate this situation successfully?* True discipline isn't about controlling your child—it's about teaching them how to control *themself.*

THE HIDDEN MESSAGES IN OUR WORDS

The words we use during moments of discipline carry significant weight, often more than we realize. Whether they're intentionally or unintentionally positive, neutral, or negative, our words become part of the "data" children use to form their sense of self. By choosing words that connect rather than criticize, you're not just transforming behavior—you're teaching your child how to navigate their emotions, repair mistakes, and grow into their best self.

Blame
- **Outward Message:** "What did you do?"
- **Hidden Message:** You're at fault.
- **Shift:** "What happened here?"
- **New Message:** Let's work together to figure this out.

Shame
- **Outward Message:** "Why did you do that?"
- **Hidden Message:** You've made a mistake, and I'm disappointed.
- **Shift:** "You're holding your sister's toy, and she's crying. What happened?"
- **New Message:** I see there's a problem, and I want to understand and help.

Guilt
- **Outward Message:** "You should know better."
- **Hidden Message:** You've failed me or let me down.
- **Shift:** "It's frustrating that I said no, and I won't let you hit me."
- **New Message:** Having big emotions is normal, and I'm here to guide you through this.

Judgment
- **Outward Message:** "That's not nice" or "Stop being bad."
- **Hidden Message:** You're a bad person because of your behavior.

- **Shift:** "You grabbed the toy your sister was playing with. It's not available because she's using it."
- **New Message:** Your actions have consequences, but they don't define you.

Fear
- **Outward Message:** "If you keep doing this, then we're not getting ice cream."
- **Hidden Message:** You need to fear losing something to comply.
- **Shift:** "Looks like you're having a hard time stopping. Let's try this instead."
- **New Message:** I see you're struggling, and I'm here to help you succeed.

The Anatomy of Effective Discipline

True discipline isn't about control; it's about *teaching*. It's about guiding your child toward self-regulation and growth. Discipline isn't something you *do to* your child—it's something you *cultivate with* them.

The word *discipline* itself comes from the Latin *discipulus*, meaning "pupil."[2] Let that sink in for a moment: True discipline is focused on learning. It's about equipping your child with the skills they need to navigate the world—not punishing them into submission.

The recipe for effective discipline—creating connection, setting clear limits, and teaching skills—is designed to move from trying to be in control to being in charge and becoming a true leader guiding your child. All three elements are equally important and can be broken down as follows:

1. **Creating Connection:** Using both physical and emotional connection helps your child feel seen and heard by meeting them

where they are—not where you want them to be. This helps you create cooperation as your child sees you on their team.
2. **Setting Clear Limits:** Clear, consistent, yet kind limits and expectations, when paired with your help to follow through on them, provide structure and create a secure environment where your child can thrive.
3. **Teaching Skills:** Discipline is about teaching your child *how* to navigate life's challenges—not punishing them for getting it wrong. Through teaching conflict resolution, emotional regulation, communication, and problem-solving skills, you equip them with the tools they need to make better choices and regulate themself.

Positive, effective, developmentally appropriate discipline empowers parenting by building trust and connection that foster mutual respect because a toddler needs to feel safe and secure to learn. Leaving fear and control behind and focusing on meeting your child where they are developmentally, not where you wish they were, allows you to work with your child's development—not against it.

Shifting Your Discipline Style

Transitioning from conventional discipline to positive, effective, developmentally appropriate discipline isn't a simple flip of a switch—it's a process. It means unlearning old habits, challenging deeply ingrained beliefs, and embracing a new way of parenting. Most importantly, it means shifting your mindset and how you interpret your child's behavior. Without this, it's extremely hard to shift your discipline style. It's not always easy, but the rewards are undeniable. Positive discipline fosters trust and strengthens the parent-child bond, which in turn creates cooperation, nurtures your child's development, and lays the groundwork for raising an emotionally healthy, resilient child.

Here are three key mindset shifts that can empower you to change discipline styles:

Mindset Shift #1: From "My Toddler Is Being Bad" to "My Toddler Is Having a Hard Time Coping"

- **Empowered Truth:** Toddlers lack the brain development and life experience needed to regulate their emotions and behavior. All behavior is communication—a way of expressing a feeling, emotion, or unmet need.
- **What to Do:** Instead of labeling the behavior as "bad," address what's driving it. Support your child through their big emotions while setting limits on unsafe or unacceptable actions.

Mindset Shift #2: From "I Need to Control My Toddler's Behavior" to "I Can Only Control Myself"

- **Empowered Truth:** Control is an illusion—you can't truly control another human being. Trying will only leave you frustrated and trigger your child's developmental need to assert their independence, creating more power struggles.
- **What to Do:** Focus on what you *can* control: your own words, actions, and responses. By modeling calm and thoughtful behavior, you set the stage for cooperation and understanding.

Mindset Shift #3: From "I Need to Teach My Toddler a Lesson" to "I Need to Teach My Toddler Skills"

- **Empowered Truth:** Effective discipline isn't about punishment; it's about teaching. Your role is to guide your child toward developing the skills they need to handle their emotions, navigate challenges, and make better choices.
- **What to Do:** Use connection, clear limits, and skill building to help your toddler learn and grow.

This kind of shift doesn't happen overnight. It's a journey that requires patience, persistence, and plenty of grace—for your child *and* for yourself. But each time you choose connection over control, each time you focus on teaching instead of punishing, you're not just influencing your child's behavior and rewiring your brain. You're creating the foundation for healthy relationships, emotional self-regulation, and resilience that will serve them throughout their lives.

Understanding Consequences

Parents and caregivers that are new to developmentally smart discipline constantly ask me, "But what consequence should I give this behavior?"

I want to be clear: **The goal here is to transform behavior through teaching skills,** *not* **punish a child for a lack of skills.**

So when it comes to teaching our children about the impact of their choices, **natural and logical consequences** are the tools we want to focus on rather than **arbitrary consequences** (which is another name for punishment). Let's break them down.

Natural Consequences

Natural consequences are the outcomes that occur naturally, without adult intervention. Children learn best through experience, and natural consequences are the universe's way of saying, "This is what happens when you make that choice."

Examples of Natural Consequences
- Running on an uneven sidewalk → Tripping and falling
- Refusing to wear a coat → Feeling cold outside

Why Natural Consequences Work
- They help kids develop decision-making skills by experiencing real-world outcomes.
- They foster a sense of control, allowing children to take ownership of their choices.
- They reduce power struggles by shifting responsibility away from the adult.
- They build confidence as kids learn to manage themselves effectively.

Using Natural Consequences Effectively
- Ensure safety first—no learning happens in a dangerous situation.
- Step back and let the consequence unfold, even if it's hard to watch.
- Help your child process the outcome and teach them skills to navigate it in the future.

Logical Consequences

Logical consequences are introduced by an adult and are directly related to the behavior in question. These are your go-tos when natural consequences aren't safe or practical. The key here is to make the consequence *relevant, respectful, and reasonable* (thank you, Dr. Jane Nelsen!).[3]

Examples of Logical Consequences
- **Scenario:** A child is throwing blocks and won't stop.
- **Response:** "Let's put the blocks away and try again later."

In this case the behavior (throwing blocks) leads to the consequence (removing the blocks).

THE THREE R'S OF LOGICAL CONSEQUENCES

1. **Relevant:** The consequence ties directly to the behavior.
   - Example: Throwing sand from a sensory bin leads to the bin being put away.
2. **Respectful:** The consequence maintains the child's dignity.
   - Example: If a child spills milk, the parent helps them clean it up rather than scolding them.
3. **Reasonable:** The consequence is fair for both the child and the adult.
   - Example: Removing blocks for the day after throwing is reasonable; banning blocks for a week is not.

Why Logical Consequences Work
- They teach self-control and responsibility.
- They maintain trust and respect between parent and child.

Using Logical Consequences Effectively
- Be proactive—set your child up for success by adjusting the environment. For example: If splashing during bath time is a problem, fill the tub with less water.
- Allow your child to try again before enforcing a consequence. "I see you are having trouble keeping the water in the tub. You can splash the back wall like this."
- From a place of curiosity, ask, *What's really driving this behavior?* Address the root cause, not just the surface action. "I wonder if you are trying to get my attention so I will play with you."

Arbitrary Consequences

Arbitrary consequences are unrelated, adult-imposed punishments designed to control behavior.

Example of Arbitrary Consequences
- **Scenario:** A child throws a toy at their sibling.
- **Response:** "That's not nice. No ice cream tonight."

In this case the consequence (no ice cream) has nothing to do with the behavior (throwing a toy).

Why Arbitrary Consequences Fail
- They don't teach anything about the original behavior.
- They create confusion and resentment.
- They rely on external control, not internal growth.

By focusing on natural and logical consequences, you're teaching your child how the world works in a way that's safe, supportive, and empowering. However, if you focus only on consequences and limits, you're missing the bigger picture. Discipline isn't about control or compliance—it's about teaching. The real recipe for effective discipline must include *all three* key ingredients: connection, setting limits, and teaching skills.

When we shift from just enforcing rules to guiding and teaching, we help toddlers develop self-regulation, problem-solving, and emotional resilience. Again, discipline isn't something you do *to* your child—it's something you do *with* them to help them grow.

TODDLER TIP
Choose Connection over Correction: Time-Outs vs. Time-Ins

When your child's behavior is out of control, use a time-in instead of a time-out. While both remove the child from the situation, time-outs are designed to isolate the child, which cuts them off from their safe and secure base (you!) when they need connection the most. Time-outs fail to address the root cause of the behavior; in other words, they're a punishment. This is why you will usually see a child's behavior escalate during a time-out.

Time-ins, on the other hand, are rooted in connection. When you remove your child from a situation and stay with them, you help them calm down, process their feelings, and move from their downstairs brain (where big emotions rule) to their upstairs brain (where they can think, problem-solve, and learn). By choosing time-ins over time-outs, you're not just correcting behavior—you're teaching your child how to regulate their emotions and handle challenging situations with resilience and grace.

Getting Your Child to Listen

Toddlers aren't mini-robots you can program for instant obedience—they're humans with developing brains. That's why the first step in getting your toddler to listen is understanding that listening isn't about compliance; it's about fostering cooperation. If you define listening as "doing exactly what I say the instant I say it," you're setting yourself up for power struggles and a lot of frustration.

Instead, shift your mindset to see listening as a dynamic relationship rather than a demand-response transaction. It's about building trust, creating influence, and fostering an environment where your child wants to work with you because they feel seen, heard, and loved.

One of the most effective ways to encourage cooperation is by acknowledging the behavior you want to see. This foundational positive-parenting strategy reinforces desirable actions while helping you focus on the positive. It's easy to get stuck noticing only the misbehavior because what you pay attention to grows.

SCRIPTS FOR COMMUNICATION
Acknowledging Positive Behavior

Positive parenting starts with seeing—and celebrating—small wins.

Try Saying

- "I saw you put your spoon in the dishwasher—thank you for helping!"
- "You handed your baby brother his rattle—that was so thoughtful!"
- "You were so upset, but you kept your hands to yourself. That took a lot of self-control!"
- "I saw you wanted to bite, but you stopped yourself—great job using your words instead!"

> Remember, acknowledging progress matters—even when it's not perfect. If your child usually hits when angry but manages to pause, recognize the effort. This reinforces that effort and improvement are noticed, building a foundation for lasting positive change.

Your toddler is wired to seek your approval because, deep down, their greatest need is for your unconditional love and acceptance and their greatest fear is losing it. They watch closely, picking up on the behaviors that grab your attention. When they sense you're excited or pleased by something they've done, it lights them up inside. They want to see that spark of joy in you again and again because feeling connected to you is their most powerful motivator.

As you tackle the daily challenges of parenting, remember that every moment of connection, every clear limit, and every skill you teach is shaping your child's ability to listen and understand—not just with their ears but with their whole being. Getting your toddler to listen is about more than just obedience; it's about building a relationship that will empower them to make good choices, even when you're not there to guide them.

At the end of the day, discipline isn't about control—it's about raising a child who can think, feel, and make good choices on their own. And that starts with how we guide them today.

TODDLER TIP
Set Clear Limits

When you ask your child to do something, avoid adding "Okay?" at the end. It makes the request sound optional, giving them the chance to say no—even when it's not a choice.

> Imagine you're at the park, and it's time to go home. Instead of saying, "It's time to leave in five minutes, okay?" you can maintain authority by getting close, kneeling to their level, and saying, "It's time to leave in five minutes. I'm setting a timer. What's the last thing you'd like to do before we go?"
>
> This approach allows you to set a clear limit while inviting cooperation.

Chapter 16

BUILDING CONNECTION

Connection is the most powerful parenting tool in your tool kit—and the *first ingredient* in the recipe for effective discipline because it goes beyond merely managing behavior. It's about building a deep, authentic relationship. By meeting your child where they are—physically, emotionally, and mentally—you allow your child to feel truly seen, heard, understood, and unconditionally loved. It helps your child see you as on their team instead of as an opposing force, which opens the door to more cooperation, which leads to influence, which in turn creates more cooperation. When your child feels connected to you, you are able to walk hand in hand with them over the bridge to where you want them to be instead of trying to drag them there kicking and screaming, or standing there expecting them to navigate their way on their own.

Connection Is Vital to Transforming Behavior

Connection is the balm that soothes emotions, helping children regain their emotional equilibrium. It's not just a powerful parenting tool—it's often the only tool needed when we're faced with challenging behavior. Connection doesn't just de-escalate big emotions; in many cases, it dissolves the behavior entirely. Here are a couple of my favorite examples of the power of connection:

Example 1: The *Bluey* Meltdown

When one of my clients decided it was time to turn off *Bluey*, her son lost it—full meltdown mode. Instead of pushing harder, repeating limits, or doling out consequences, she leaned into connection.

She sat down beside him, stayed calm, and said, "I know you really don't want to turn off *Bluey*. You love this show sooo much. You wish you could watch it forever."

Through tears and shouts of "No! I don't want to!" she kept holding space, reflecting his feelings back with deep empathy: "I know, buddy. You're having so much fun, and stopping feels really hard."

After what felt like an eternity—but was really only about five minutes—he let out a big sigh and said, "Yeah, I know." Then he got up and turned off the TV.

No power struggle. No bribes. No punishments. Just connection.

Example 2: The New-Baby Struggle

My friend Becky had just welcomed a new baby into the family, and her toddler was struggling with the transition. He wanted his mom to put him to bed instead of his dad, but she was nursing the baby. Instead of resorting to logic or a firm limit—"I'm sorry, I can't. Your dad is putting you to bed"—Becky chose connection.

She sat with him and said, "I know. It's so hard having a baby sister. She needs so much care and can't even play with you. Instead, she just cries and takes up so much of our time."

She let that sink in. She didn't rush to fix it, didn't try to change his feelings. She just sat with him in that truth.

After a long pause—what felt like an eternity—her toddler softened, nodded, and walked off to his room without protest.

Many parents fear addressing the "elephant in the room"—the thing their child is already thinking and feeling—worried that saying it out loud will make things worse. But more often than not, the opposite is true.

Toddlers, just like adults, want to feel seen, heard, and understood. When you name their internal experience, you show them you're on their team. You help them process and make sense of what's happening and how they feel about it.

Now, I'm not saying this will magically work every time, but more often than not, it will soften the behavior—and that's a game changer.

Creating Authentic Connection

One of the biggest mistakes parents make when it comes to fostering connection is expecting instant results just because they said the right words. I often hear from parents who feel frustrated: "I told my child, 'It's okay to be upset, but you need to listen to me.' But my child was still upset and crying." Just because you went through the motions of connection doesn't mean your child feels connected.

> ### TODDLER TIP
> *Instead of* But, *Use* And
>
> After you connect with your toddler and validate their feelings, use *and* instead of *but* before you set the limit or expectation. Why? Because you connect with your child and support them in feeling seen, heard, and loved through validation. When you follow that validation up with *but*, then set a limit or expectation, it tends to invalidate what was said before *but*—as though your agenda is more important than their feelings, needs, and wants. However, *and* can serve as a bridge between the two

> sides. When a child feels connected to their caregiver, it creates influence, and influence creates cooperation. There is a distinct difference between "You are having so much fun playing *but* it's time to leave" and "You are having so much fun *and* it's time to leave."

The truth is connection isn't about saying the magic phrase or checking a box. It's about showing up—fully present and patient—even when your child's response isn't immediate. Connection means slowing down, pausing, and being willing to make more than one attempt. Because connection isn't transactional; it's relational. It's not something you "get done" so you can quickly move on to setting limits or teaching skills. Children need to *feel* that you are with them, not just hear reassuring words.

So when your child stays upset after your first attempt, consider it an invitation to try again—not a failure. Take a breath, meet them where they are, and try another way. Offer comfort through touch, use a calming tone, or sit quietly with them if that feels right. Real connection is built moment by moment—not rushed, not forced, but deeply felt.

The Two Faces of Connection

Let's break down connection into two essential types: **physical** and **verbal**.

Physical Connection

Think of physical connection as the gateway to your child's heart. It's the look in your eyes when you meet their gaze, the gentle touch of your hand on their shoulder, the way you crouch down to their level so you can see the world through their eyes. Physical connection is letting them know that they matter, that they're seen, valued, and safe, by practicing some of the following actions:

- **Creating Proximity:** Coming alongside your child instead of talking across the room increases your ability to connect with your child and be heard.
- **Getting on Their Level:** Physically lowering yourself to your child's height changes the dynamic. You're no longer the towering authority figure; you're approachable, meeting them where they are. This invites openness and trust.
- **Touch:** A reassuring hand on their back, a hug after a meltdown, holding hands as you walk together—these gestures are powerful, nonverbal ways to connect. They say, "I'm here. You're safe. We're in this together."
- **Eye Contact:** When your child talks to you, look them in the eyes. This simple act conveys that you're fully present, listening not just to their words but to the emotions and thoughts behind them. Remember, don't force eye contact, as it can be too intense for some kids.

> **TODDLER TIP**
> *Prioritize Physical Connection First*
>
> Create physical connection with your toddler so you have their attention before you start talking to them—especially when you are asking them to do something.

Verbal Connection

Verbal connection is where the magic happens. This type of connection is about creating a safe space for your child to express themself, and to know that you're there to understand them. It encourages connection through the words you choose and the tone of your voice, particularly when you approach your child with the following strategies:

- **Observe and Describe:** Before responding to your toddler's behavior, take a moment to observe what is happening. Then describe it out loud in a neutral way like you are a reporter: "You are running around when I asked you to put on your shoes."
- **Curiosity:** All behavior is communication, and it's our job to get curious and uncover the root of behavior. Plus, it helps your toddler feel seen and heard as you become a teammate instead of an opposing force. Approaching your child with genuine curiosity opens the door to understanding and cooperation. So instead of jumping to conclusions, ask questions like these:
    - "I wonder if . . ."
    - "What's your plan?"
    - "What happened here?"
    - "How can we make this better?"
    - "How can I help you?"
    - "What made you want to hit?"
    - "What are you trying to tell me?"

  This not only helps you uncover the feelings, emotions, and needs at the root of their behavior but also shows your child that their thoughts and feelings are worth exploring.
- **Validation:** Validating your child's feelings, emotions, and experiences doesn't mean you agree with or condone their behavior. It helps your child feel seen, heard, and understood. Validate their feelings, even if you don't agree with their actions. An easy way to do this is to say, "I hear you saying . . ." then repeat back what they said. You can also say, "How frustrating that your sister took your toy, *and* I won't let you hit." Even a simple acknowledgment can be incredibly powerful in helping your child feel understood: "You were so mad you wanted to bite."
- **Authentic Empathy:** Meet your child where they are emotionally. If they're sad, be sad with them. If they're excited, share in their

excitement. Empathy doesn't mean solving their problems; it means being with them in their emotions, showing them that they don't have to go through it alone.

- "I remember feeling like this too."
- "Some days I don't want to leave the house either."
- "It's hard to share Mommy with the baby."

- **Playfulness:** This is the most underused and underrated parenting tool, and it's one of the quickest ways to connect with your toddler and get them on your team because play is the language of toddlerhood! This looks like giving a piggyback ride to the bathroom at bath time or letting them stand on your feet and walking them to the door. Practice putting logic aside and connect with your ability to be playful.

> **TODDLER TIP**
> *Make Time for Connection*
>
> Set aside ten minutes per day of distraction-free, one-on-one time with your child with the sole purpose of following your child's lead and delighting them. That means putting away your cell phone and letting your child be in charge. Follow their lead and give them your focus.

Connection isn't just a parenting strategy—it's the heart and soul of raising a child who feels loved, valued, and understood. Whether it's getting outside to explore together, sharing your daily highs and lows, or giving your child positive attention, when you prioritize connection (along with the rest of the recipe for effective discipline), you're not just shaping your child's present moment but also laying the foundation for a lifetime of secure, healthy relationships. A secure attachment is formed when your child knows they can rely on you to be there, both physically and emotionally, no matter what. This is the anchor your child will return to, time and time again, as they navigate the world. So lean into it. Meet your child where they are, with open arms and an open heart, and watch as they blossom in the safety of your connection.

Chapter 17

SETTING LIMITS

The second step in the recipe for effective discipline is setting clear, consistent, and firm—yet kind—limits. Limits aren't just rules; they're the guardrails that help your child navigate the world. By now, you know that toddlerhood is all about your child figuring out who they are—separate from you. They're testing, pushing, pulling (and yes, sometimes driving you up the wall). But through limits, toddlers learn essential life skills: emotional regulation, frustration tolerance, and how to manage their behavior within a safe, structured environment.

In fact, limits help your child feel secure. When toddlers have too much power, it can actually feel overwhelming—like they're steering a ship without a map. They need a sense of control and autonomy, but they also need to know that you're in charge. Predictable limits create a sense of safety, while consistency and follow-through reduce power struggles over time. When a child knows what to expect, they're less likely to push back because they trust that you mean what you say.

Know Your Role

One reason it can feel so hard to set limits is because we aren't clear on our role in the process. Without clear limits, we can easily slip into being the Permissive Pushover. You might be parenting from the Permissive

Pushover role if you rarely set limits or you usually don't follow through and often give in when your child screams, cries, or pushes back against the limits you set.

However, if we focus solely on setting limits and gaining compliance but forget about connection and teaching skills, then we tend to slip into the role of the Controlling Commander.

Here's the deal: It's your job to set the limits. It's your toddler's job to test them. And they will. That's not them being difficult—it's them doing exactly what they're supposed to do as they figure out how the world works and where they fit within it.

Your Job	*Your Toddler's Job*
Set limits.	Test limits.
Follow through on limits.	React to limits.
Support your toddler's emotions.	Accept limits.

It's completely normal for your toddler to have a big emotional reaction when they hit a limit because it challenges their sense of control. That might look like kicking, crying, or screaming. It's not defiance; it's processing. Your job isn't to stop the reaction but to stay calm, consistent, and compassionate as they work through those big feelings.

So what do you do when your toddler looks you straight in the eye and says no? First, take a deep breath. This is developmentally appropriate behavior. In fact, a toddler's first instinct is often to say no—even when they actually want what's being offered. Pause for a moment, and you might be surprised when they change their mind.

If that doesn't happen, resist the urge to use punishments, bribes, or threats. Instead, focus on connection and curiosity. Try saying, "I hear you saying no. I wonder if you want to keep playing?" or "What's your idea?" Sometimes a little partnership or a shift in approach is all it takes to turn resistance into cooperation.

TODDLER TIP
Disrupt the Cycle

If you ask your child to do something two or three times and they still aren't listening or keep saying no, then it's time to disrupt the cycle and try a new angle. This usually means you need to increase your level of physical and/or emotional connection with your child. So move closer, get down on their level, place a hand on their shoulder, and try again. If they are still struggling, then you need to help them follow through. For example, if you ask your toddler to stop pulling the dog's tail and they don't stop, go kneel beside them and try again. If they still don't stop, then move the dog or your child to help them follow through: "I see you are having a hard time stopping. I won't let you pull his tail." Then you move your child or the dog.

Setting Limits Successfully

Okay, we know limits are important. But how can we ensure they are *effective*? Let's dive into what makes a limit truly effective, and how you can master the art of setting them. Here are some practical tips for setting limits:

- **Set Expectations in Advance:** Toddlers thrive on predictability. Let them know what's coming before a transition or change. For example, you might tell them: "We are going to the store. We won't bring home any toys today, but we can look at them." Setting expectations helps them mentally prepare for what's next, and sometimes we forget to do this because we assume a child knows what is next or what is expected. The more you communicate, the better.

- **Be Clear and Concise:** Less is more when it comes to setting limits. Keep your tone neutral and your words simple. Toddlers need us to stand firm while still being kind and taking their needs and emotions into account.
- **Create Connection:** Toddlers are less likely to listen if you are talking to them from across the room. Get close and create connection by putting your hand on their shoulder or kneeling beside them before setting the limit.
- **Give a Warning:** Transitions can be tricky for toddlers. Giving a five-minute warning before setting a limit gives them time to adjust. "In five minutes, we'll put the toys away. I'm setting the sand timer so you can see." This small gesture can make a big difference in cooperation.
- **Follow Through:** Only set limits you are willing to follow through on. Toddlers are little scientists, always testing the limits and looking for the weak link. Once they find it, they'll keep pushing until you give in or they know you are serious. If you're not willing to follow through, it's better not to set the limit at all. Consistency is key so your child knows your words have integrity.
- **Partner with Your Child:** Think of limits as a team effort. Work together to meet the limit rather than punishing them for failing. "I see you are having trouble petting the dog gently like this. I'm going to move the dog away to keep everyone safe."
- **Create a Win-Win:** Find ways to meet your toddler's needs within your boundaries. When your toddler is jumping on your new couch, say, "It looks like you want to jump. Let's jump on the play couch or trampoline." This way, your toddler feels heard, and your limits stay intact.
- **Take the Lead:** One of the most disempowering traps we can fall into is waiting for our child to comply instead of confidently taking the lead. When we wait for our child to decide whether to comply, we inadvertently invite them to question the limit or even ignore it altogether. This can erode the sense of consistency and predictability that helps them feel secure. For example, it's time to brush their teeth, but they're resisting. Head to the bathroom, turn on a fun song, and start brushing your own teeth, modeling the behavior you want to see.

SCRIPTS FOR COMMUNICATION
Setting Limits Confidently

Scenario
   Your toddler is splashing in the dog's water dish.

Try
- **Connect:** Start by acknowledging what is happening and your toddler's feelings and needs. "There's water on the floor. Looks like you were playing in the dog's water dish. You love playing in water."
- **Limit:** Clearly state the boundary in a neutral tone. "The dog's water stays in the bowl."
- **Teach:** Offer a solution that respects both your boundary and your toddler's need. "Looks like you want to play with water. Let's fill the sink with water and play."

Preserving the Power of No

No is a powerful word—for both you and your child. But as parents, we often find ourselves on the defensive, firing off *no* after *no*, only to watch in frustration as our toddler throws it right back—or does the exact opposite of what we asked. And who could blame them? Toddlers are wired to seek independence, and hearing *no* over and over can trigger their natural drive to push back and assert control.

They're also learning by imitation, and *no* is one of the few tools they have to express their budding autonomy. And it's actually important for toddlers to practice saying no. It helps them build confidence in setting boundaries, a skill they'll need for the rest of their lives.

TODDLER TIP
Don't Overuse the Word *No*

Toddlers are like little mirrors that reflect our words and actions. The more you say no, the more your toddler will say no—and the more you yell, the more your toddler will yell. *No* is best reserved for moments of danger and unsafe behavior, such as running toward the street or biting another child.

Okay, so why not just say no when your toddler asks for something unreasonable or when they do something "bad"? Because *no* is a brick wall. It stops the conversation dead in its tracks. It can trigger your child's developmental drive for independence and cause a meltdown or power struggle. But offering a path forward—now that's a door that opens to possibility. It turns a *no* into a *not yet*.

TODDLER TIP
Turn a *No* into a *Not Yet*

When your child wants something and you need to set a limit, turn the *no* into a *not yet* by telling your child the next time they can do or have the thing they want—or give them a choice within your boundaries. It reduces power struggles because it gives your child something to look forward to instead of having them hit a brick wall.

Using this tip, if your child wants a cookie, instead of saying, "No. We don't have cookies for breakfast. That's not healthy," you

> might try, "You really want a cookie. You love them! You can have one for a snack today. Do you want it for a morning snack or afternoon snack?"

Toddlers need limits to thrive. It's okay to tell your toddler no—you just don't want to overuse it.

Overcoming Challenges in Setting Limits

Setting limits confidently takes practice. Here are some common challenges parents run into and how to overcome them:

Challenge 1: Consistency

Consistency isn't about perfection; it's about predictability. A lack of consistency with limits will increase limit-testing behavior. If you falter, don't stress—just course correct. If you set a limit then change your mind, don't freak out. If it happens, do your best to course correct without reinforcing their protesting.

Example: Your toddler asks for a banana but you are about to make lunch. You say no and start making lunch, and your toddler has a full-scale meltdown. You realize they are hungry and need to eat now. "The more I think about it, you must be really hungry. Let's sit down at the table and have a banana appetizer while I finish making your lunch."

Challenge 2: Following Through

Toddlers often need help to meet an expectation due to their lack of impulse control and developmental drive to test limits as they strive to understand how the world works.

Example: Your toddler starts throwing sand out of their sensory bin. You calmly say, "I see you're throwing the sand. Sand stays in the bin." When they throw it again, you follow through: "I see you're having trouble keeping the sand in the bin. It's time to take a break, and we can try again later." Then you put the sand away. *Later* could be five minutes later or five weeks later. If they become upset, you stay neutral and supportive: "I know you're upset. You love playing with sand. I'm here to help."

Challenge 3: Navigating Big Emotions

Your toddler's big emotions can be overwhelming, but they're a normal part of development. Don't shy away from them. Stay grounded, take care of your own needs, and practice responding intentionally rather than reacting. Accept all emotions as valid, even the uncomfortable ones. Your calm presence teaches them how to weather emotional storms.

Example: It's time to leave the park, you've already given a five-minute warning, and your toddler is now refusing to go, shouting at the top of their lungs, "No!" Kneel next to them and say calmly, "I hear you. You don't want to leave because you're having so much fun. It's hard to leave, isn't it?" Pause and let that sink in before continuing. "We'll come back again soon." Then, you set the limit: "It's time to go now." Offer a choice: "Would you like to walk to the car, or should I carry you?" When they don't choose and continue to protest, stay neutral. "Looks like you're having trouble deciding. I'll help you get to the car." Pick them up gently, prepared for their big emotions, and offer reassurance: "I know this is hard. I'm here with you."

Remember, it's not your job to make your child happy. It's your job to keep them safe and teach them skills. Sometimes they won't like what you have to say, and that's okay. What's important is that you support their big emotions while still following through on your word.

Toddlers are little scientists, and they are going to test limits. Limits provide the structure within which your toddler can safely explore the world. By setting effective limits with clarity, empathy, firmness, and consistency, you're not just transforming behavior—you're nurturing a secure, confident little human.

TODDLER TIP
Tell Them What to Do (Not What Not to Do)

Did you know toddlers often miss the meaning of negative sentences like "No jumping on the couch"? They tend to focus on the action itself, hearing only "jumping on the couch." To avoid this, frame instructions positively:

Instead of: "No standing on the chair."
Say: "Chairs are for sitting. Your feet stay on the floor."

Instead of: "Don't throw food."
Say: "Food stays on your plate."

Instead of barking orders, pause, think about what you want them to do, and communicate that clearly. And, yes, you might have to show them what you mean—literally. "No running!" becomes "Let's walk beside the pool," and sometimes that means taking their hand and leading the way if they need help following through.

Chapter 18

TEACHING SKILLS

The last step in the recipe for effective discipline is teaching skills. Every behavior challenge is an opportunity for learning—for both you and your child. Think about it: Every time you teach your child how to handle their emotions, solve a problem, or navigate a tricky situation, you're setting them up to handle those challenges on their own in the future. Instead of infinitely having to step in to fix things or mediate every conflict, you're equipping them with the tools to take ownership of their behavior and decisions. Yes, positive, effective, developmentally appropriate parenting takes more effort up front, and your toddler won't master these skills overnight. Yet teaching skills to your toddler is the ultimate way of working yourself out of the job of parenting—*because the true goal of parenting isn't just to manage behavior but to foster independence and confidence that will carry them through life*.

The ultimate success in parenting isn't to raise a child who constantly needs us to step in but to raise one who can navigate the world with resilience and self-reliance.

We can practice and teach our children the following skills:

Social Skills / Conflict-Resolution Skills

Think of yourself not as a referee who steps in to blow the whistle and dole out penalties but as a coach in the long game. When conflict arises—whether it's name-calling, a push, or a toppled tower—addressing it is not just about determining who's right or wrong. It's about guiding your toddler to understand the impact of their actions, take ownership, and learn how to repair relationships, which are all essential skills for their future.

Strategies to Foster Social Skills / Conflict-Resolution Skills
- **Use "I" Statements:** Teach your toddler to take ownership of their feelings by modeling simple phrases like "I feel _____ when _____ because _____." For example, "I feel sad when my tower gets knocked down because I worked hard on it." These statements help them communicate their emotions and needs more effectively.
- **Make Amends:** Guide your toddler through the process of repairing relationships when they've hurt someone (see chapter 38, "Modeling Manners"). For example, "Your sister is crying because her tower got knocked down. How can you make it right? Maybe you could help rebuild it."
- **Embrace Disagreement:** Teach them that it's okay to disagree and show them how to do it respectfully. For instance, if one child wants to play dolls and the other doesn't, you might say, "You want to play dolls and your sister doesn't. You don't always have to agree."
- **Teach Through Modeling:** Remember that your actions speak volumes. Every time you apologize, resolve a disagreement calmly, use respectful language, or make space for someone else's feelings, you're modeling these skills and what it means to handle differences with empathy and grace.

Emotional-Regulation Skills

Big, messy emotions—anger, frustration, sadness—are part of being human, especially for toddlers who are just learning how to navigate their feelings. And when these big feelings show up, it can feel like your patience is hanging by a thread. But here's the magic: Every meltdown or moment of frustration is an opportunity to teach emotional regulation. Every deep breath, every empathetic response, and every narrated moment is another building block in your toddler's emotional toolbox. And as they practice, they'll grow into someone who can weather the storms of life with resilience and calm—a skill that starts with you.

Strategies to Foster Emotional-Regulation Skills
- **Model Grounding Techniques:** When you feel overwhelmed, take a pause and narrate what you're doing to calm yourself. Try saying, "I'm feeling frustrated, so I'm going to take some deep breaths to help myself calm down." Later, reflect with your toddler: "Remember earlier when I felt upset? I took deep breaths. Let's practice together."
- **Give Them Simple Strategies:** Help your toddler practice calming techniques. For example, say, "Next time you feel angry and want to hit, you can squeeze your hands together like this" (then demonstrate making a fist). Practicing these techniques together helps them feel more natural when big emotions hit. (For more ideas, see chapter 19, "Calming an Upset Toddler.")
- **Narrate Real-Life Situations:** Everyday moments are perfect teaching opportunities. If you're at the playground and see another child crying because it's time to leave, point it out to your toddler: "Looks like she's crying because it's time to go, and she doesn't want to. I wonder if she feels sad. Sometimes we cry when we're sad." This kind of narration helps your child connect emotions to actions and understand that feelings are valid and manageable.
- **Validate Their Feelings:** When your child is in the middle of an emotional storm, acknowledge their feelings. Say, "You didn't like that your sister grabbed your toy. It's unsafe to push your sister. Let's find a safe way to tell her you're upset." This teaches them that emotions are natural and acceptable, but unsafe actions are not acceptable.

Communication Skills

Toddlers are in a phase of rapid language development, often referred to as a "language explosion." During this time, teaching them how to communicate effectively can significantly reduce frustration and prevent tantrums. By giving your child tools to express themselves, you're helping them navigate their world more confidently.

Strategies to Foster Communication Skills
- **Expand Their Vocabulary Through Books:** Reading together is one of the best ways to help your child build their vocabulary,

and research show that kids who are read to more have immensely bigger vocabularies.[1] As you read, point out words, ask questions, and connect the story to their experiences. For example, if a character looks sad because they lost their toy, you could say, "Oh no, they look sad. They lost their favorite toy. Have you ever felt sad like that? What did you do?" This encourages your child to recognize emotions in themself and others while practicing how to express their own feelings.

> For a helpful list of my favorite books, visit transformingtoddlerhood.com/bookresources.

- **Use the Body to Communicate.** Show your toddler how to use their body to communicate. For instance, teach them to hold up their hand and say "Stop" when a sibling or peer is invading their space. Simple physical gestures like this can empower them to set boundaries and express themself clearly.
- **Use Baby Sign Language:** Introducing signs for basic needs like "eat," "water," "more," and "help" can reduce frustration and give your toddler a way to communicate before they've fully mastered their expressive-language skills. This can also help decrease tantrums caused by communication breakdowns.

And as always, model the tone you want your toddler to use—kind, firm, respectful. They'll mimic what they hear, so make sure what they're hearing is what you want them to repeat.

Problem-Solving Skills

You don't have to have all the answers. And, spoiler alert: You don't have to solve every problem. When it comes to teaching problem-solving skills, the most important thing is helping your toddler to think through and navigate the little puzzles life throws their way. You're creating a partnership, where you're not just the fixer but the guide, the mentor, the cocreator of solutions.

Oftentimes, things that we think are problems actually aren't—they are just typical toddler behaviors and reactions. Your toddler isn't broken and doesn't need to be fixed. In fact, sometimes the best thing you can do is step back, giving your toddler space to work through a challenge with your support if needed.

Strategies to Foster Problem-Solving Skills

- **Get Curious:** Encourage your child's curiosity and critical thinking by asking questions like "What can you do next time?" or "How could we make this better?" or "Now can you tell me you are mad without hitting?" Then help your child practice a more skillful response.
- **Brainstorm Together:** Treat challenges as opportunities for collaboration. For example, if they're struggling to reach a toy, ask, "What could we use to get it?" If they don't have an answer, offer suggestions to get their ideas flowing, such as, "Maybe a stool? Or could you ask for help?" It can also be helpful to give your child a choice between two options that are within your boundaries.
- **Celebrate Imperfect Solutions:** Not every solution will be perfect, and that's okay. Let your child try their idea, even if it's not ideal. If it doesn't work, use it as a teaching moment: "Hmm, that didn't work the way we thought it would. What else could we try?" This helps them build resilience and confidence in their ability to problem-solve.

Putting It into Practice

The number one key to teaching new skills? Timing. Teaching skills is best done in a calm moment—once a child is regulated and back to their emotional equilibrium—not in the heat of the upset. When your child is upset and overwhelmed, their brain is in "downstairs mode," which means they're not in a place to learn and practice new skills. Trying to teach in these moments will backfire.

Instead, focus on practicing skills during calm, connected moments. These moments help build the "muscles" for using the skills when challenges arise. Once they've practiced in a calm setting, they'll be better equipped to try them in harder situations. Better yet, use play as a tool for teaching skills, making the learning process enjoyable and engaging. For example, use animal figurines or dolls to role-play different scenarios to help your toddler practice social and problem-solving skills in a fun way.

Teaching skills should also be collaborative—something you do *with* your child, not *to* them. If your toddler is younger and unable to respond when you ask a question or offer guidance, that's okay! They're still taking in much more than you realize. In these cases, come up with a way to move forward and model it for them. Even if they're not able to use words yet, your actions and modeling lay the foundation for future learning. Once they're older, the process will already feel familiar and natural to them.

Teaching skills isn't a one-time event—it's a continuous process, woven into the fabric of daily life. You are planting seeds that will grow into skills your child will use for the rest of their life. It's about taking those everyday moments, the meltdowns, the squabbles, the frustrations, and transforming them into opportunities for growth. It's about equipping your toddler with the tools they need to navigate the world, to build relationships, to solve problems, and to regulate their emotions.

Part 3

THE EMOTIONAL TODDLER

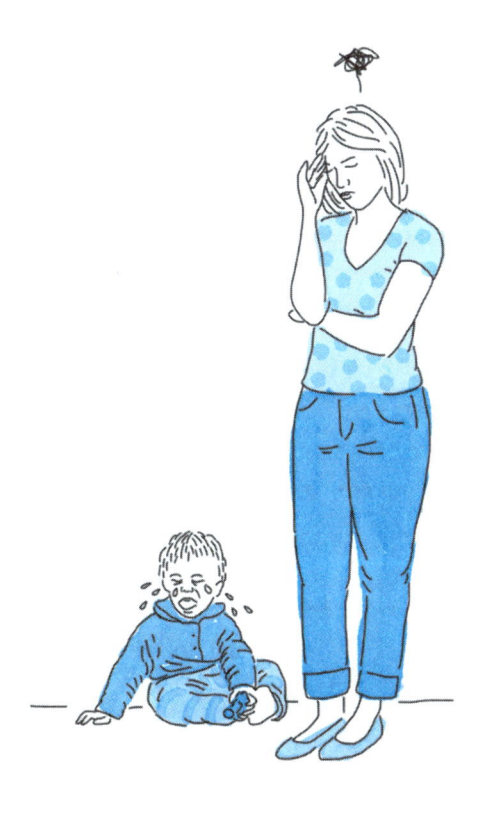

Chapter 19

CALMING AN UPSET TODDLER

Imagine this: You're hungry and tired, but you don't have the words to explain how you're feeling. Or maybe you know the words but can't access them right now because you are too overwhelmed and upset. The discomfort builds, turning into frustration, and you try to communicate the only way you know how—through sounds, actions, and tears. The more overwhelmed you feel, the harder it becomes to manage. You want to say something, but the words simply aren't there. Frustration bubbles up, and it's so overwhelming that you scream and flail, trying to release the feelings building inside you—only to be met with someone yelling at you to stop, right when you're starting to feel a little better.

Toddlers become dysregulated by all types of emotions and sensory experiences. Excitement and anticipation can unravel a child just like frustration, anger, and jealousy. Another child might be overwhelmed by a loud indoor play gym or an inconveniently placed tag in their clothes. Dysregulation can look different for every child, ranging from a serious case of the sillies to running around the house to crying and screaming on the floor.

For toddlers, the world can be a confusing and overwhelming place, filled with unmet needs, unfamiliar expectations, and emotions too big to handle alone. And for parents, navigating these emotional storms can feel just as challenging. Dealing with a dysregulated toddler is physically draining and emotionally exhausting.

Big Emotions Are for Everyone

Here's a truth every parent needs to hear: It's completely okay for your toddler to have big emotions—and it's okay for you to have them too.

Emotions aren't good or bad; they just are. Yet many of us grew up being taught, directly or indirectly, that some feelings are "good" and others are "bad." This conditioning often sneaks into our parenting. When our children's big emotions make us uncomfortable, we might try to fix them, make them stop, or shut them down entirely.

Feelings are signals that give us insight into our children's internal landscape. Like the weather, they can be stormy sometimes, and sometimes calm, a passing rainstorm coming and going. Toddlers, in particular, live so fully in the moment that once the storm passes, they often bounce back to their sunny selves pretty quickly.

Of course, this emotional resilience is harder to maintain when your child has unmet needs—when they're tired, hungry, sick, sensorily overwhelmed, traveling, or navigating big life changes like starting school, adjusting to a new sibling, or dealing with a family transition. These challenges can wear down their ability to recover quickly from emotional upsets.

And that's okay too. This messy, unpredictable process of feeling, expressing, and recovering is part of what makes us human. Embrace it—it's a beautiful opportunity to teach your child that all feelings are welcome and manageable.

All Emotions Are Valid

Far too often, toddlers are punished, shamed, or ignored for having developmentally appropriate behavior and reactions. But they don't need punishment. *They need our support.*

Your toddler's frustration over a peeled banana, their sadness about heading to daycare, or their devastation when their favorite show ends? It's no less real than your feelings of longing for life pre-kids or the frustration that creeps in when bedtime stretches on forever.

With our fully developed brains, we tend to look at toddler behavior through a lens of logic and think, *Ugh, they're making such a big deal out of nothing.*

Just because it doesn't seem like a big deal to us doesn't mean it's not a big deal to your child. We need to switch to an emotional lens, not a logical one.

AVOIDING POSITIVE DISMISSIVENESS

We can accidentally dismiss feelings in an attempt to make a child feel better. It can be uncomfortable to encounter the full spectrum of emotions from your child. The more you can expand your capacity for this, the more you can make the biggest difference in your child's life when they are having the hardest time.

So instead of saying, "You're okay" or "It's not a big deal" when your toddler is upset, try saying one of these:

- "That was disappointing."
- "This is really hard."
- "I hear you."
- "That was really _____ [scary, sad, etc.]."
- "I hear that you need space. I'll stay close by."
- "Tell me about it."
- "I'm here with you."
- "I will help you work it out."
- "I'm listening."

At the same time, as parents and caregivers, we often push *our* emotions aside. We let everyone else's feelings take center stage, ignoring our own until frustration, anger, and resentment bubble over.

Here's the truth: Your child's feelings matter just as much as yours. Everyone's emotions hold equal weight.

The big difference is that adults have tools (both positive and negative) to help us manage our big emotions—things like going for a run, eating chocolate or a tub of ice cream, drinking alcohol, crying, screaming into a pillow at the top of our lungs, calling a friend or a therapist to vent. Yet the most important tools we possess are a fully mature brain, lots of life experience, and a large amount of control over our lives.

Toddlers? Not so much. When they're hit with those same big emotions, they lack the brain development and coping tools to handle them. So they do what they *can* do: They cry, yell, whine, hit, throw things, or scream.

That's why they need you—not just to comfort them but to help them learn how to navigate all the intense emotions bubbling up inside. It's not your job to make your toddler happy, but it is your job to allow your toddler to experience the full spectrum of emotions and guide them through.

The Art of Co-Regulation

The best way to help your toddler calm down isn't by telling them to calm down; it's to find your *own* calm first.

At the heart of helping toddlers manage their emotions is something called **co-regulation**. Co-regulation is the process through which a caregiver or trusted adult provides emotional support and guidance to a child, helping them manage and regulate their emotions during moments of stress or dysregulation. It involves the adult maintaining or regaining their own calm and using that calmness to soothe the child, modeling emotional regulation and gradually teaching the child how to manage their emotions independently. Co-regulation is a critical part of early emotional development because young children, particularly toddlers, do not yet have the neurological capacity to self-regulate on their own.

Toddlers are often more attuned to their caregivers' emotions than we give them credit for. There's even a name for this phenomenon:

emotional contagion—the process by which one person's emotions can spread to another, particularly in close relationships. Research shows that a parent's emotional state can significantly influence a child's mood and behavior.[1] That means if you're stressed or anxious, your toddler is likely to pick up on those feelings and mirror them, which can exacerbate their own emotional struggles. This is why practicing maintaining your own calm during a toddler meltdown is so crucial—not only are you modeling emotional regulation, but you're also providing a stable emotional environment for your child to find their own calm.

TODDLER TIP
Start with Self-Regulation

Focus on calming yourself down first before addressing your child's behavior. A dysregulated adult will struggle to calm a dysregulated toddler. While you model calming yourself down, your toddler may start to calm down as well. To assist with this, use techniques from the Calming Plan in chapter 8 ("Becoming a Safe Parent").

Most parents feel the pressure to have it all together, to keep their emotions in perfect check, but that's just not realistic. You're going to lose your patience because you're a human being with your own feelings, emotions, needs, and triggers. You're going to have moments when your own big emotions get the better of you. And guess what? That's okay too. What's important is what you do next. When you model how to bounce back and regulate yourself as well as repair the relationship by making amends (see chapter 8, "Becoming a Safe Parent"), your child is learning these essential skills right alongside you. The sooner you accept your big emotions, practice creating calm within yourself, and model this for your toddler, the sooner they'll learn to accept their own big feelings. This is the foundation of self-regulation—a skill they'll carry with them for life.

CO-REGULATION IN ACTION

Actions That Support Co-Regulation	Actions That Do Not Support Co-Regulation
modeling calming down	blaming your child for your feelings
sitting near your child during a tantrum	yelling at or punishing your child during a tantrum
checking on your child during a tantrum	ignoring your child during a tantrum
allowing your child to release their feelings and emotions	using fear, coercion, and threats to create compliant behavior
reassuring your child of your love and that they are safe	shaming your child for not being able to regulate their emotions and behavior

Toddler Fears

Children first start to understand a fearful experience around eight to twelve months old, but more complex fears start to emerge around two years old. These fears can range from the dark to loud noises to the thought of being separated from you, and they can feel overwhelming and unmanageable to a little one. The good news is that fear is a normal part of development. As toddlers begin to make sense of the world around them, they also start to feel anxiety without yet having the tools to manage it.

Addressing these fears doesn't have to be overwhelming. Here's a five-step guide to help you navigate them:

1. **Acknowledge the Fear Without Dismissing It:** Instead of brushing off your toddler's fear or telling them there's nothing to be afraid of, validate their feelings and experience. For example, "You don't like the bugs on the sidewalk. I'm right here. Why don't we step back and watch where the bugs go?" This lets them feel seen and heard and know that you're there to support them.
2. **Stay Calm and Neutral:** Your reaction sets the tone for how your child perceives the situation. Staying calm shows them that fear isn't something to panic over. For instance, if your toddler is afraid of the closet door being open, you could say, "You don't want the closet door open at night. I'll look inside with the light on—would you like to come with me? Then we'll turn the lights off together. You are safe."
3. **Celebrate Small Moments:** When your child faces a fear, even in a small way, recognize their effort. After they try something that once scared them, like the big slide at the park, you might say, "You were nervous about going down the big slide, and you did it!" Acknowledging their courage builds their confidence.
4. **Create Positive Experiences:** Introduce new experiences that foster joy and curiosity in a way that feels safe. If a specific experience sparked the fear, like a negative interaction with a dog, work on creating positive associations. Start with small, safe exposures—watching a calm dog from a distance, looking at pictures of dogs, or playing with stuffed animal versions. Or, for example, if your child is scared of water, start with playful, low-pressure interactions like splashing hands in a small tub or playing with toy boats. Positive experiences help reshape their perspective.
5. **Use Imaginative Play to Process the Fear:** Imaginative play allows toddlers to work through their fears in a safe, controlled environment. Role-playing scenarios with dolls, puppets, or toys can help them process their emotions. For example, act out a scenario where a stuffed animal confronts a similar fear. Reversing roles—where your toddler plays the adult and you play the child—can also empower them by giving them a sense of control.

Ultimately, your child needs to know they're not alone in their fears. By staying calm and supportive, you teach them that fear is manageable, and they can rely on you for guidance. This foundation of trust and openness will grow with them, helping them feel secure and resilient as they navigate their emotions.

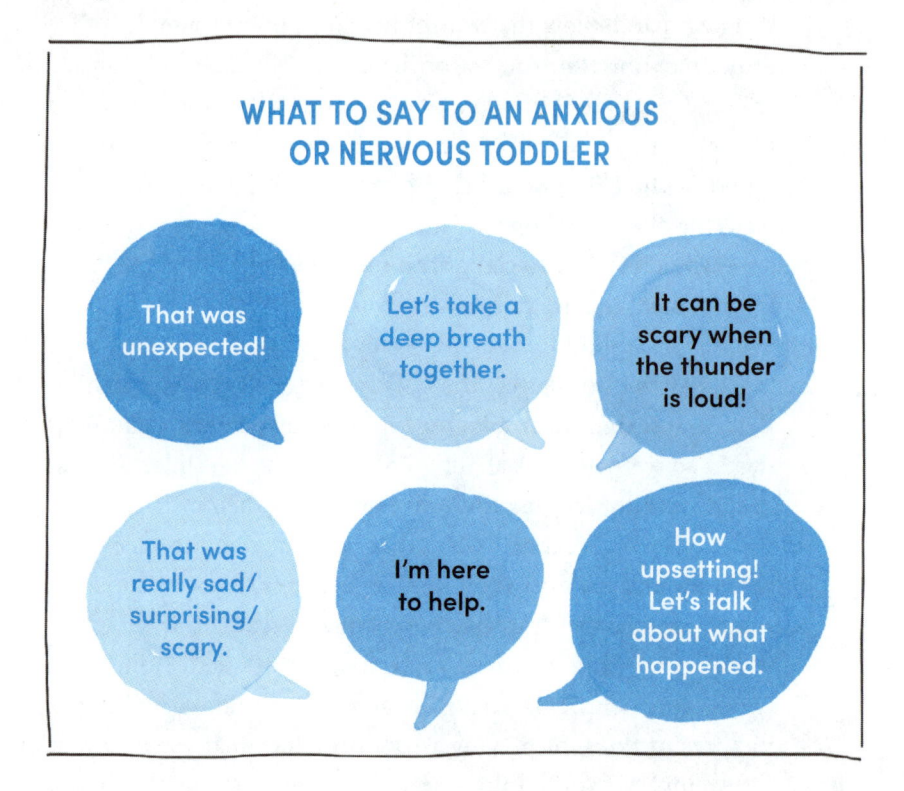

WHAT TO SAY TO AN ANXIOUS OR NERVOUS TODDLER

- That was unexpected!
- Let's take a deep breath together.
- It can be scary when the thunder is loud!
- That was really sad/surprising/scary.
- I'm here to help.
- How upsetting! Let's talk about what happened.

Practical Strategies for Calming an Upset Toddler

When your little one is dysregulated, your goal is to provide a calm presence, to be the anchor in their storm so you can help your child process and move through their feelings, getting them back to their emotional equilibrium. This might mean sitting quietly with your child, offering a comforting touch, or simply letting them know that you're there when they're ready. It's about holding limits without holding a grudge, and about showing your child that their big feelings are okay—that they are okay, even when they're struggling.

> ### TODDLER TIP
> *Practice Calming Skills in Advance*
>
> Teach your child calming skills in the calm moments—not when your toddler is in full meltdown mode. These are the times when your toddler's brain is most receptive to learning new ways to handle big emotions. In those moments of dysregulation, your child's brain isn't ready to learn. They're in survival mode, and the part of their brain responsible for logic, reasoning, and learning is offline. Imagine being completely overwhelmed with emotions, your brain screaming *fight* or *flight*, and someone is trying to give you a lesson on how to stay calm. It wouldn't work for you, and it doesn't work for your toddler. Toddlers need lots of practice in the calm moments to later be able to access these skills in the challenging moments.

There are several practical, connection-based strategies and calming tools that will help you guide your child through the storm rather than being swept away by it. Keep in mind these tools aren't meant to be used all at once and are organized into ones you can use in the moment of chaos and others for calmer times. You can do one or several. Practice these calming techniques as part of your daily routine, such as before bed or after your toddler's nap.

During the Chaos: Tools for Staying Calm and Holding Space
- **Model Your Own Calming Tools:** Remember, your calm is contagious. Your toddler looks to you for cues on how to respond to their environment. If you practice staying calm during stressful

situations, they're more likely to mirror that calmness and learn those skills.

- **Breathe Audibly:** Practice deep-breathing exercises, and when your toddler is upset, invite them to breathe with you. Instead of saying, "You need to calm down right now. You're out of control!" try saying, "This is hard. Let's take a couple of deep breaths together and figure this out." Don't force your child to take deep breaths. Take them yourself and they may or may not follow. Even if they don't do it, calming yourself will help them calm down too.
- **Verbalize Your Calm-Down Process:** When you're feeling frustrated or overwhelmed, narrate your own process of calming down. For example, say, "I'm feeling upset, so I'm going to take a few deep breaths and count to ten to help me feel better."
- **Use a Calming Corner or Calming Kit:** Set up a dedicated calming area in your home with soft pillows, favorite stuffed animals, some quiet toys (such as bubbles and a fidget popper), and books. This space should be inviting and associated with peace.

> For more ideas on how to do this, visit transformingtoddlerhood.com/bookresources.

- **Go Outside:** Nature can be very soothing and regulating, especially for young kids.
- **Whisper:** Using a soft voice can help you stay calm and soothe your child.
- **Hold Space for and Acknowledge Feelings:** When your toddler is upset, let them express their feelings without trying to fix them. Validate their emotions by saying things like, "I see you stomping your feet. I wonder if you are feeling mad."
- **Offer Physical Touch:** Physical touch can be incredibly soothing. A gentle hug, holding hands, or simply sitting close can help your toddler feel secure and loved. You can also use your hands to give firm, deep-pressure "squeezes" to your child's shoulders, arms, legs,

and feet, or give your child a weighted blanket to help calm their nervous system.
- **Create Forward Momentum:** If you always wait for your toddler to calm down completely before moving on, you might unintentionally fuel their tantrum by giving the undesirable behavior too much attention. Redirecting their focus can help de-escalate the situation while still supporting your child's emotions. This could look like turning on their favorite song, changing environments by going outside, or just moving on to the next task to help your toddler move on from the upset.

During the Calm: Tools to Teach and Practice Calm

- **Read Books Together:** Books are a great tool for teaching toddlers and help increase their emotional literacy.

> For my curated and up-to-date list of my favorite social/emotional skills books, visit transformingtoddlerhood.com/bookresources.

- **Practice Identifying Emotions:** Hang an emotions chart on the wall that shows facial expressions for different emotions. Then use a mirror to practice making facial expressions to match emotions. If your toddler is resistant, focus on modeling this activity. They are still learning even if they don't participate.
- **Listen to Meditations Together:** Teaching children about meditation early in life can support their emotional well-being for the rest of their lives. Research has shown that meditation can increase gray matter in areas of the brain responsible for emotional regulation, learning, and memory.[2] There are several apps and audio players that can facilitate this, or you can create a meditation and lead yourself and your child through it.
- **Practice Breathing Techniques:** Breathing is a powerful tool that we can use to calm our nervous system when we are in a stress response. Here are a few of my favorite techniques:

- **Candle Blowing:** Have your toddler hold up a finger and exhale slowly, pretending to blow out a candle.
- **Belly Breathing:** Your toddler can lie on their back and watch their belly go up and down while they inhale and exhale. You can even place a stuffed animal or toy on their belly so they can watch it go up and down.
- **Smelling a Flower:** Have your toddler pretend they are smelling a flower and practice inhaling through their nose and breathing out through their mouth.
- **Tracing a Hand:** Teach your toddler to breathe while tracing your hand or their hand, inhaling at the top of a finger and exhaling when they drop between two fingers.
- **Bubble Blowing:** Let your toddler practice blowing bubbles. You can do it, too, modeling breathing in through your nose and out through your mouth to blow the bubbles.
- **Counting Breaths:** Inhale slowly for two to three counts, then exhale slowly for three to four counts. Focus on making the exhale longer than the inhale.

• **Teach Sensory Strategies:** Understand your child's sensory preferences. As they get older, partner with them to learn which type of sensory input (or lack of input) helps them feel calm, and have those tools available for them. For example, I have noise-reducing earmuffs on a hook at my toddler's height. He can put them on when I turn on the blender or when there are other sounds that feel overwhelming and dysregulating to him. Or have a swing available if swinging is calming for your child. There are many other types of sensory input you can use based on your child's needs to calm them. (Please refer to chapter 12, "Getting to Know Your Toddler's Sensory System.")

Every parent wants to raise an emotionally healthy toddler. Just because your toddler is a big ball of emotions now doesn't mean they won't grow up to be emotionally healthy. What matters is how we respond to them and the tools we teach them.

Toddlerhood can be messy—physically and emotionally. Don't be afraid of messes. They happen, and just like spilled milk or scattered toys, they can always be cleaned up. Remember that every tantrum, every overwhelming emotion, is an invitation—an opportunity to connect, to practice, and to grow. Not just for your child but for you too. So the next time your toddler's tears start to flow, take a deep breath. Ground yourself in the knowledge that this is part of the process and embrace the chance to guide your child through the storm with love and confidence.

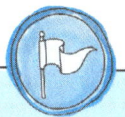

RED FLAG
Ongoing Emotional Dysregulation and Outbursts

If your toddler is constantly going from one upset to another, or it seems like a dark cloud is hanging over them for days and weeks at a time, or their emotional outbursts are completely derailing the family and everyone is walking on eggshells, this is cause for further investigation with your pediatrician or other child professional, like a pediatric occupational therapist or play therapist.

FAQs

I tried to validate my child's feelings and now they are even *more* upset. Why did this happen and what do I do?

When a child becomes more upset when you try to connect and validate their emotions, it can mean three things:

1. **They Feel Safe Enough to Off-Load Their Emotions:** Your child trusts you, so they're releasing all the pent-up emotions they've been carrying. This release can intensify their upset feelings before

they return to emotional balance. In this case, slow down. Hold space for their emotions by staying calm and present. Keep validating their experience and offering comfort—whether through hugs, soothing words, or simply being there.

2. **They Are Highly Sensitive and Feel Overwhelmed:** Sensitive children may experience embarrassment or shame about their intense emotions or behavior. In these cases, validating their feelings might feel overwhelming, causing them to escalate further or even lash out physically. When this happens, step back and give them space to calm down. Once they're regulated, revisit the situation and focus on narrating what happened rather than analyzing their emotions in detail.

3. **They're Unsure About Your New Approach:** If your response style has changed—for example, if you've shifted from yelling to calm validation—they may feel uncertain and test whether this new response is consistent and genuine. They're gauging whether you can handle their big emotions and behaviors without reverting to old patterns. In this case, stay steady. Keep validating their feelings and fostering connection, showing them through your actions that your calm, supportive approach is here to stay.

My child is running around the house laughing and being completely out of control. I told him to stop, and he won't. What's going on?

This is a sign that your child is dysregulated. It's important to meet your child where they are instead of trying to demand they do what you want. One way to handle this is to join them by running with them or engaging by directing their running. For example, you might say, "You really want to run! Okay, do a lap around the couch. Now the chair." This playfulness and connection can create enough influence to move them on to the next things. Another way is to move on to the next thing in your agenda and give your child some space. They will likely come find you when they realize you have moved on. You can also employ some of the techniques from the sensory chapter (chapter 12) to help get their nervous system regulated.

I have three kids who all feed into one another's energy, and before I know it, they are all bouncing off the walls or all three of them are crying. How do I handle this?

As long as everyone is safe, start by addressing the child who seems most receptive to your support in the moment. Once that child is calm, shift your focus to the next one who appears ready to engage. If their behaviors are unsafe, prioritize creating physical safety—try doing something unexpected to redirect their attention or separate the children if needed. Once safety is established, focus on calming them down.

Chapter 20

TRANSFORMING TANTRUMS

Toddlerhood and tantrums often go hand in hand, like thunder and lightning—unpredictable, loud, and sometimes a little scary. One moment, your sweet, giggling toddler is a bundle of joy, and the next, they've morphed into what feels like a tiny tornado of emotion, flailing, crying, and completely inconsolable.

Your child isn't a little monster when they're in the throes of a tantrum. They're simply a toddler—a tiny human trying to navigate a big world with an emotional tool kit that's still very much under construction.

Tantrums happen when your toddler's emotions or sensory system becomes too overwhelming and they aren't able to express what they need, want, or feel with words. Intense emotions like anger, fear, frustration, or disappointment can flood them, triggering an automatic stress response in their lower brain.

At this point, your toddler is stuck in their emotions, unable to regulate or calm themself. The crying, screaming, or other outbursts you see are their way of communicating just how overwhelmed they feel on the inside. These behaviors may seem chaotic, but they are an honest reflection of emotions that have become too much for them to manage.

The Truth About Tantrums

Tantrums are a typical part of development from ages one to four, peaking between eighteen and thirty-six months, and are essential for your child's emotional growth. As frustrating as they can be for both you and your child, tantrums play a vital role in helping your little one learn to manage their feelings and, in turn, behavior, while cultivating resilience. They're an emotional release, not a sign of a bad child or bad parenting. When the world feels too big, too fast, or just too much, a tantrum is the body and brain's way of saying, "I need help."

The good news? By the time your child hits five, tantrums usually begin to subside, unless they've been unintentionally reinforced or if there's a developmental or sensory challenge at play. But knowing that tantrums are typical doesn't always make them easier to deal with. What helps is understanding the underlying message behind the overwhelming outburst.

TANTRUMS VS. MELTDOWNS

While I use *tantrum* and *meltdown* interchangeably throughout this book, understanding the difference between the two can help you respond more effectively. In the toddler years, the lines often blur because toddlers are still developing emotional-regulation skills, and their brains are far from fully mature. For this reason, both tantrums and meltdowns can be developmentally appropriate during this stage.

Tantrums

- Tantrums are emotional outbursts that can be physical or verbal.
- They are often **goal-oriented (strategic)**, typically aimed at getting a need or desire met, such as wanting a toy, snack, or connection.

- Tantrums usually subside when we consistently don't give in to them—unless your child has an unmet basic need like being hungry, tired, or overstimulated.

Meltdowns
- Meltdowns are also physical or verbal outbursts but are **not goal-driven**.
- They happen when a child is overwhelmed by emotions, unmet needs, or sensory overload.
- Meltdowns tend to end when the child exhausts themself or when a parent provides calming support to help them regulate.

When a tantrum is unsuccessful it can sometimes turn into a meltdown.

Tantrums Are Communication

Every behavior is a form of communication, and your child's tantrum is no different. It's their way of saying, "I'm overwhelmed" or "I don't know how to cope with this." Understanding what your child's behavior is trying to tell you can make all the difference in how you respond.

Here are some common messages and triggers behind tantrums:

- **Overwhelm or Frustration:** They may be feeling out of control and lacking the physical or verbal skills to express themself.
- **Struggling to Cope:** They may find it difficult to manage big emotions, physical sensations, or limits set by others.
- **Desire for Change:** They may be attempting to alter something in their environment, often in the only way they know how.
- **Unmet Needs:** They may be reacting to unmet physical, emotional, sensory, or developmental needs.

- **Sensory Overstimulation:** They may be overloaded by sensory input, leading to a meltdown.
- **Not Getting Their Way:** They may express frustration when their desires or expectations aren't met.

REFRAMING TANTRUMS

The key to responding effectively to tantrums lies in how you view and relate to them.

We can do this by applying the following mindset shifts, which are similar to the ones we learned in chapter 15 ("Redefining Discipline"):

Mindset Shift #1: From "My Toddler Is Being So Bad Right Now" to "Aw, My Toddler Is Having Such a Hard Time Right Now"

- **Empowered Truth:** A child's behavior doesn't make them good or bad. That's a judgment we impose on the behavior. Instead, recognize that at the root of all behavior are feelings, emotions, needs, and desires. Your child isn't misbehaving—they're struggling to manage big emotions.

Mindset Shift #2: From "This Is a Problem to Make Go Away" to "This Is a Learning Opportunity for Us Both"

- **Empowered Truth:** Tantrums can feel like a problem when we resist accepting developmentally appropriate behavior—usually because it triggers something in us. However, each tantrum is an opportunity for learning, both for you and your child. Children need chances to fall apart in a safe space with a supportive adult to learn how to regulate themselves.

> *Mindset Shift #3: From "My Child Is Being Manipulative" to "My Child Is Being Strategic to Get Their Needs Met"*
> - **Empowered Truth:** If your child has learned that tantrums are an effective way to get what they want or avoid what they don't, it doesn't mean they're manipulative. It means they're clever and resourceful in trying to meet their needs.

Responding to Tantrums

When your child has crossed the threshold into a full-blown tantrum, trying to stop it is like holding back a rushing river—it doesn't work and only increases frustration for both you and your child. Plus, suppressing the emotional release can cause emotions to build up even more, leading to bigger outbursts later.

Instead, focus on helping your child ride the emotional wave and release their emotions. Falling to pieces and then coming back together is a critical part of learning how to self-regulate. Your role is to meet your child where they are emotionally and guide them back to calm—not force it.

Your primary goal during a tantrum is to help your child move from their "downstairs brain" (emotional, reactive) to their "upstairs brain" (rational, regulated). This means meeting them at their level of dysregulation and offering a safe, calm presence until they're ready to reconnect. Think of the tantrum like a bell curve. You're more likely to connect with your child as they ramp up or wind down, not at the height of their emotional storm.

Tantrums are *not* the time to

- reason or explain (your child isn't in a place to process logic),
- punish or shame (this only heightens their distress), or
- force your child to calm down (it's a process, not a command).

While it's natural to want to avoid or stop a tantrum, trying to do so can often backfire. When we try to prevent a tantrum by giving in or appeasing our children, we might unintentionally reinforce the behavior, which can make tantrums happen more often and for longer.

That said, some days, you may not have the energy to ride out a tantrum, and you might find yourself giving in. This doesn't make you a bad parent—it makes you human. The key is consistency, not perfection. Consistency means that more often than not, your response is predictable, which creates a sense of safety and trust for your child.

And if you've unintentionally reinforced tantrums in the past, it's never too late to shift gears. With consistent limits and a calm, supportive approach, you can help your child learn healthier ways to express their emotions and get their needs met. Remember, you're not aiming for perfection—you're aiming for progress.

A Step-by-Step Approach to Responding to Tantrums

Here is a framework to help you respond to tantrums more effectively:

Step 1: Ensure Safety

- **Physical Safety:** Make sure both you and your child are in a safe environment. Move to a safer space if needed or set firm limits to prevent harm.
- **Emotional Safety:** Take deep breaths, stay calm, and remind yourself that this is not an emergency. Focusing on staying calm is the most powerful thing you can do during a tantrum once your child is safe. Your steady presence is essential for your child's regulation through co-regulation.

Step 2: Create Connection

- **Follow Their Lead:** Pay attention to how much connection your child can handle during a tantrum. Sometimes less is more.
- **Address Their Physical Comfort:** Offer a hug or sit close by if they're receptive.

- **Offer Validation and Reassurance:** Use calm, validating statements like "You didn't like that" or "I'm here to help" or "You really wanted more muffins." Less is often more at the height of a tantrum.

Step 3: Uphold Limits
- **Stick to Limits:** Maintain the original limit that triggered the tantrum to avoid reinforcing the behavior.
- **Address Unsafe Behavior:** Calmly but firmly set limits around actions like hitting or throwing: "I won't let you hit." Don't try to physically restrict your child by holding their hands. This can make your child more upset. Instead, move away from them or put a pillow or cushion between you to help them follow through.
- **Use Simple, Consistent Language:** Keep your words clear and predictable even if it takes longer than you want it to.

Step 4: Embrace Emotions and Wait It Out
- **Allow Emotional Release:** Let your child express their feelings without judgment.
- **Stay Calm:** Your calm presence helps them feel safe enough to work through their emotions.

Step 5: Move Forward and Teach Skills
- **Reassure and Reconnect:** Offer reassurance and help them return to a regulated state.
- **Offer Choices:** Provide simple, age-appropriate options to give them a sense of control.
- **Teach Skills:** Once they are calm, discuss better ways to handle similar situations in the future or work together on problem-solving.
- **Track Behavior:** Pay attention to patterns—what time of day tantrums happen, what triggers them, and what your child might need in those moments. Tracking can help you prevent future tantrums. Use this information to anticipate and potentially prevent future

tantrums by addressing underlying needs, such as hunger, tiredness, or overstimulation.

> ### TODDLER TIP
> *Take the Lead*
>
> Instead of waiting for your child to make the first move, take the lead in moving forward. The other day, my child really wanted a mango bar from the pantry. I let him know he could have another tomorrow, which upset him, and he ended up on the floor crying. The longer I stayed and engaged, the more intense his crying became—because he still had hope I might change my mind.
>
> Rather than staying in a standoff, I turned on some music and started setting up his train set nearby. Within minutes, he asked for his plate of food and came to sit near me to eat and play.
>
> Taking the lead doesn't mean ignoring your child's emotions—it means acknowledging their feelings while gently guiding them toward the next moment. This approach teaches them that while their emotions are valid, life keeps moving forward, and new, positive experiences are always waiting.

You've Got This!

Navigating tantrums is no small feat, but with a positive mindset and developmentally appropriate strategies, you can turn these challenging moments into opportunities for growth—both for you and your child. Remember, perfection isn't the goal; consistency and patience are. Each tantrum is a chance to practice, learn, and strengthen the bond between you and your child.

THE EMOTIONAL TODDLER

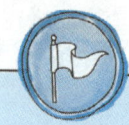

RED FLAG
Continuous Tantrums

If tantrums haven't started to decrease by age five, it may indicate that tantrums have been unintentionally reinforced and have become a preferred communication tool or that there could be underlying developmental or sensory concerns. For guidance on whether your child's outbursts fall outside the typical range of frequency, duration, or intensity, refer to these red flags from Andy Belden, a researcher at Washington University:

- Aggression toward caregivers or objects in at least half of their most recent tantrums
- Self-injury during tantrums (biting or scratching themselves, banging their head against a surface)
- Frequent tantrums (exceeding ten or twenty per month at home or more than five per day on multiple days outside the home)
- Very long tantrums (consistently exceeding twenty-five minutes)
- Inability to calm themselves or bounce back after a tantrum[1]

NAVIGATING THE PRESSURE OF PUBLIC TANTRUMS

Public tantrums can feel like one of the most dreaded parts of toddlerhood. That sinking feeling of panic and embarrassment when your toddler starts to melt down in public is something nearly every parent and caregiver experiences. You're not alone. The fear of judgment and shame can unravel even the most steadfast parent.

Here's what you need to know.

- **Human Nature Is Curious:** People will almost always stop and stare. Even if it's just out of curiosity, it can feel like judgment.
- **You Should Focus Only on What You Can Control:** You are in control of yourself and your responses. Other people's judgments only have power if you let them. People's reactions aren't about you; they stem from their own experiences. A child's tantrum can trigger emotions in others based on their own past experiences. We often interpret others' behavior as judgment when we're already judging ourselves. Practice compassion for everyone involved (yes, even that judgy onlooker—we never know what challenges of their own they may be dealing with).

Four Things to Keep in Mind During a Public Tantrum
1. **Don't Take It Personally:** Your child's tantrum isn't a reflection of you as a person or of your parenting.
2. **Shift Your Perspective:** Instead of thinking your toddler is "trying to cause a scene," understand that they're having a hard time coping.
3. **Manage Onlookers:** You have the choice to ignore them or respond with objectivity and compassion. A simple "I'm doing my best" can go a long way.
4. **Manage Overwhelm:** If at any point a public tantrum feels too overwhelming, it's perfectly fine to step away to a quiet space with your child, allowing them to work through their emotions while giving yourself a moment to ground. This might mean abandoning your cart at customer service or in the aisle and stepping outside or going to the car to calm down.

Remember, you and your child are both human and doing your best.

FAQs

Should I ignore tantrums?

Plenty of well-meaning people will tell you to ignore the tantrum to show your child this is *not* an effective way to get what they want. However, this is not developmentally appropriate. My advice is to ignore the behavior, not the child. This means that you ignore the undesirable behavior and don't play into it. However, you hold space and support your child's big emotions while helping them move through them and move on.

My toddler is hitting their head on the ground during a tantrum. What should I do?

Many toddlers will bang their heads on the ground during a tantrum in an attempt to release frustration or because they are so deep in a stress response and their nervous system is so dysregulated that they can't control their body. It's your job to keep your child safe, and here's how to respond:

Instead Of: "Oh my goodness! You are hurting yourself. Stop! Stop! Stop! This is so dangerous."

Say: "I won't let you hit your head. I'm going to keep you safe," then put your hand between their head and the floor or wall. You can repeat the action as often as needed until your child is on the other side of the tantrum or stops hitting their head.

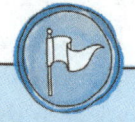

RED FLAG
Self-Injury

If tantrums are violent and self-injury escalates, then this is a red flag and a sign to speak to your pediatrician and seek extra support.

My toddler screams at me to go away, but when I do, they scream for me to come back. What should I do?

This is a sign of the contradictory emotions toddlers experience as they try to balance their need to be independent with their need for connection and emotional support. Your child may be upset at you and want some space—but at the same time you are their emotional anchor and source of comfort. They have competing needs. So give your child distance without completely leaving. Stay calm and hold space for these big emotions.

Is it okay to distract my toddler during a tantrum to make it stop?

Using a screen, treat, or giving in to demands that are outside of your boundaries and the limits you set to prevent a tantrum can reinforce tantrums. Using a screen to distract your toddler is not a solution for stopping tantrums and can lead to bigger behavior challenges later. Research has found that using media to soothe emotions and create emotional regulation is associated with "more problematic media use and more extreme emotions when media was removed in toddlers."[2] (See chapter 26, "Navigating Screen Time Confidently," for more.)

What punishment should I give my toddler if they have a tantrum?

Your first instinct might be to punish your child when they have a tantrum because you want to make it stop, and perhaps this is how your parents handled your tantrums. The truth is, punishing a toddler for having a developmentally appropriate behavior is not going to make that behavior go away. Punishing a child for a tantrum sends the message that it's not okay to feel and release their emotions. This teaches kids to shove their feelings down and ignore them. Your job is to stay calm and help your child move through their emotions and get back to their emotional equilibrium—not punish them for having big feelings.

What if I have more than one child and I can't sit with my tantruming toddler until they calm down?

It is challenging when it feels like all your children need your attention at the same time. Or if your toddler is having a tantrum while you are in the middle of cooking dinner. You don't have to stay by your child's side during the entire tantrum. It's okay to tend to the needs of the other kids and do other tasks. Here's what you can say: "I know you're upset. I'm going to the kitchen to stir the soup and I'll be back to check on you."

Chapter 21

UNDERSTANDING CRYING

Crying is a natural and essential part of a toddler's development, often sparked by moments that seem insignificant to us but feel earth-shattering to a child. This week alone, I've had parents tell me their toddler's tears have flowed for the following reasons:

- I wouldn't let the dog drive him to daycare.
- The bath was "too wet."
- He wanted syrup for breakfast—no pancakes, no waffles, just syrup.
- His sister kept "looking at him."
- He was offered a tangerine.

These tears might seem dramatic or even comical, but for a toddler, they're *deeply* real. Toddlers do not just cry for no reason. Crying isn't an overreaction—it's their way of expressing emotions too big for their little bodies and minds to handle.

So it's time we shift the way we think about crying.

Crying isn't *bad*. Crying is *healthy*.

Crying is as vital to a toddler's emotional well-being as breathing is to their body. Those tears? They're communication in its rawest, most honest form. Behind those tears is a message, and it's our job as parents to hear it.

Crying is a perfectly normal and developmentally appropriate way for toddlers (and even adults!) to release emotions and express their needs. It's their way of saying, "I need help" or "I'm overwhelmed."

At this stage of development, your child's emotional world is vast, intense, and often overwhelming. Just like babies use crying to communicate, toddlers—especially before they've fully developed expressive language—use crying, often paired with physical behavior, to get their message across. Toddlers are masters at finding the most effective way to communicate, which often means going straight to what gets the fastest results: crying plus flailing arms.

Here are just a few of the many reasons toddlers cry:

- hunger or tiredness
- trying to accept a limit
- adjusting to changes in their environment
- expressing unmet needs
- releasing stress, big feelings, fear, or emotions
- experiencing physical discomfort or pain
- feeling overstimulation or overwhelm
- seeking comfort and connection

To us, the cause of their tears might seem trivial, but that's because we're looking at it through the lens of a fully mature brain, one capable of logic and self-regulation. A young child, however, has very little control over their world and lacks the brain maturation and life experience to manage their emotions. Crying is how they cope with their feelings and process their experiences, including their lack of control in a situation. It's a crucial step in their ability to accept limits.

So don't be surprised if you set a limit or personal boundary and your child cries—it's part of the process. And sometimes those tears aren't even about what just happened. What happened might simply be the final straw, tipping the scale and opening the emotional floodgates.

We live in a culture that often values stoicism and emotional control, sometimes to a fault. This mindset can trickle down into our parenting, leading us to believe that a "good" child is one who doesn't cry, or at least doesn't cry much. But the reality is that crying has numerous emotional and physical benefits, including calming the parasympathetic nervous system, reducing stress levels, and releasing hormones that lessen physical and emotional pain.

Allowing your child to cry and then helping them navigate their emotions fosters resilience. They learn that it's okay to feel sad, angry, or frustrated and that these feelings are temporary and manageable with the right support.

How You Respond Matters

Think about the last time you just needed to cry. You felt that knot in your chest, that heaviness behind your eyes. Imagine someone telling you to "stop crying" or dismissing your feelings with "You're fine."

Brutal, right? Toddlers feel the same way—except they don't yet have the tools to regulate or articulate those emotions. They're looking to you to help them make sense of their chaos.

So when your toddler cries, imagine how good it feels to have someone sit beside you, hold your hand, and say, "I'm here. Let's figure this out together." Be that person for your toddler.

And yet, it's so easy to fall into the trap of common automatic responses. Sometimes we just want the crying to stop because it's hard to see our children so upset and we believe that if the tears end, the sadness will disappear too. Or maybe we don't think the reason for the crying is "a big deal." It's tempting to tell them to stop, to brush it off, or to rush them through it. But brushing off those feelings sends the message that their emotions don't matter.

This is where we can step in with curiosity and care. Instead of dismissing their tears, support your child through them.

Imagine your toddler is running on the sidewalk and they fall down and start crying. In an effort to comfort them, you might say, "You're fine. Don't cry." This doesn't make you a bad parent. However, what your child really needs to hear is: "You fell down. I'm here to help. Where does it hurt?"

Give them the space to express their feelings in their own way. By doing so, you're sending a powerful message: "I trust you to tell me the truth. I care about what's making you upset. Your feelings matter." These moments of connection may feel small, but they're laying the groundwork for something much bigger.

SCRIPTS FOR COMMUNICATION
Responding to Crying

Avoid Saying: "Be quiet!"
Try Saying: "It looks like you're having a hard time. I can help you."

Avoid Saying: "Stop crying."
Try Saying: "That's so disappointing. Do you need a hug?"

Avoid Saying: "You're fine."
Try Saying: "I'm right here. I know that was hard."

When you validate your child's feelings, you're telling them: "I see you. I hear you. You're safe here." And sometimes just your presence is enough.

So the next time the tears start, remind yourself that your toddler is crying because they *need to cry*. You can trust your toddler.

Show up for them. Be their anchor. And know that through every tear, you're teaching them the most profound lesson of all: They are loved, they are safe, and it's okay to feel.

UNDERSTANDING CRYING

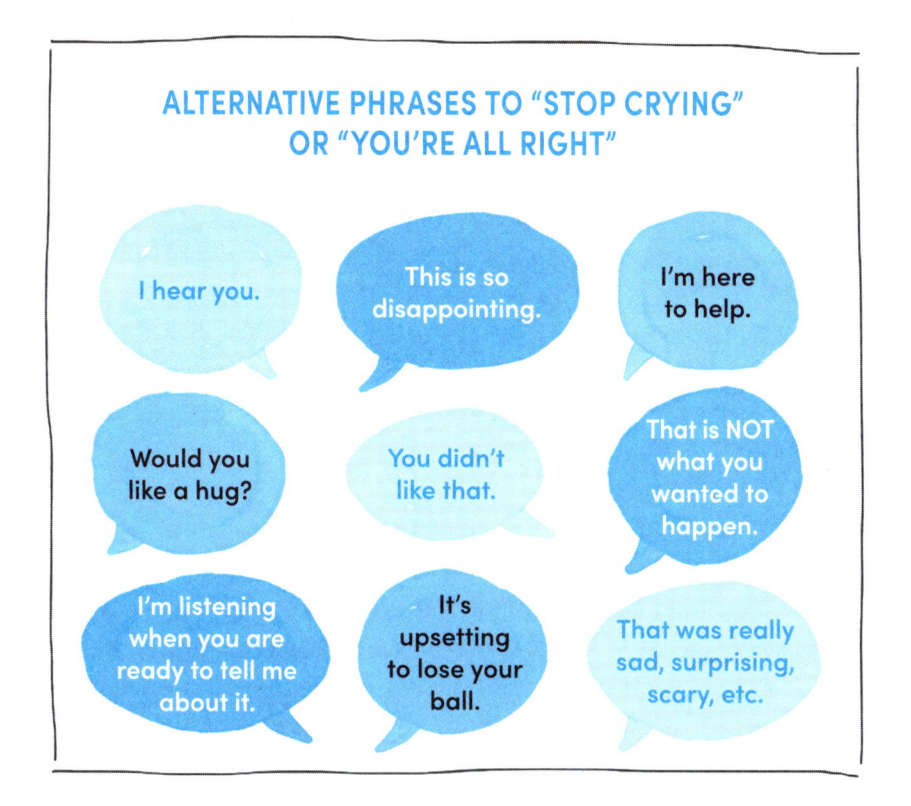

ALTERNATIVE PHRASES TO "STOP CRYING" OR "YOU'RE ALL RIGHT"

- I hear you.
- This is so disappointing.
- I'm here to help.
- Would you like a hug?
- You didn't like that.
- That is NOT what you wanted to happen.
- I'm listening when you are ready to tell me about it.
- It's upsetting to lose your ball.
- That was really sad, surprising, scary, etc.

Embrace the Tears

As parents, it's natural to want to protect our children from pain and discomfort. But when it comes to crying, the best thing we can do is lean into the experience with them. If you want your child to feel safe coming to you with life's *big* problems later on, you need to first show up for the *small* ones. Every time you validate their feelings, every time you listen, every time you help them navigate their emotions, you're building a foundation of trust and emotional safety. These little moments are how you show them that they are always seen, always heard, and always loved.

And as you embrace the reality of tears, you're not just helping your child navigate their emotions; you're helping them build the emotional resilience that will carry them through life.

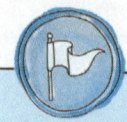

TODDLER TIP
Fake Crying Does Not Exist

It's easy to feel frustrated when your toddler's tears seem to come "out of nowhere" or appear to be an attempt to "get their way." But here's the truth: There's no such thing as fake crying. Every tear your child sheds is communicating something, even if it's not immediately clear to you. Remember: Toddlers are strategic, *not* manipulative.

What might seem like manipulation is often your child's way of expressing a need or emotion they don't yet have the words for. Maybe they're testing limits, seeking connection, or struggling to accept a situation. Whatever the reason, those tears are a call for connection, not dismissal. Crying is their way of saying, "I'm overwhelmed. I need help."

FAQs

My toddler constantly cries when she doesn't get what she wants. What should I do?

It's tough being a toddler. It's a moment in time when they have a developmental drive to have a sense of control, but they actually have very little control over their lives. So it can feel devastating to them to not get what they want. Focus on finding opportunities to give your toddler a sense of control within your boundaries when it's appropriate for your family.

Is it okay to cry in front of my toddler?

Many people are afraid to cry in front of their kids. Crying in front of your child makes you a strong leader in showing what it means to be human. Of course, you don't need to give your child every detail of why you are crying and shouldn't put responsibility for your emotions on them. Focus on giving developmentally appropriate information: "I feel sad right now and I'm crying. I miss Grandma."

Why does my toddler come home from daycare/school and fall apart crying? What am I doing wrong?

You're not doing anything wrong. If their teacher tells you they're fine all day, but the moment they're home, the tears start flowing over everything, it's a reflection of how much they trust you. It's hard for toddlers to hold it together all day, meeting expectations and having so little control over their world. Home, and being with you, is their safe haven—a place where they can finally let their guard down and release the emotions they've been carrying. Those tears aren't a sign of failure; they're a sign of a secure attachment. When kids cry after being away from you, it's because they feel safe enough with you to be their full, authentic selves.

Chapter 22

DECODING SCREAMING, YELLING, AND DEMANDS

Toddlers are like emotional fireworks—ready to burst with every spark of frustration, excitement, or overwhelm. Their brains are still under construction. This means toddlers respond to the world in raw, unfiltered ways, slipping into their "lower brain" when things feel too overwhelming to handle. With little impulse control or emotional-regulation skills to lean on, they navigate their emotions and their lack of control over their lives the only way they know how: through loud reactions—yelling, screaming, and demanding their way through the chaos of being so very small in such a big world.

Why Toddlers Yell

Understanding that your toddler's outbursts are part of their developmental journey can help you approach these moments with empathy—but let's be real: Knowing *why* doesn't make the *what* any easier to handle. Their drive for independence and to get their needs met often shows up as fiery impatience, and their demands erupt with the intensity of a fire alarm: "Mom! Right here!" they shout or "Snaaaack, now!" or all of a sudden everything you do is met with a shriek. It's exhausting, and the strain can quickly unravel your patience as it takes a heavy toll on your nervous system.

> **Common Reasons Toddlers Yell**
> - They're experimenting with their voice.
> - They're experimenting with our reaction.
> - They want to feel seen and heard.
> - They've learned it's effective in getting their needs met.
> - They're copying you.
> - They're overstimulated or overwhelmed with emotions and cannot cope.
> - They lack language skills.
> - They're expressing and releasing feelings like excitement or anger.
> - They lack brain maturation and self-control.

And here's where it gets even trickier: It's tempting to pacify your child just to end an undesired behavior. However, when you do this you might unintentionally be teaching them that their screaming and yelling is a powerful tool to get what they want. Every time you respond to yelling with immediate compliance, your child's brain takes note. What begins as a desperate plea for connection or a toy or a snack becomes a learned strategy, a go-to method for getting what they want. Over time, this can escalate into more frequent and intense demands, creating a challenging cycle that's hard to disrupt.

Here's how screaming, yelling, and demands can get accidentally reinforced:

- **Rushing to Stop the Noise:** Every time we give in to yelling or screaming just to make it stop, we teach our toddlers that this strategy works. Their brain logs the connection: yelling = results.

- **Labeling the Child:** When we say things like "You're being so bad!" a child starts to identify with that behavior, which can reinforce it.
- **Having Big Reactions:** It's challenging not to react with "Be quiet!" when screaming is piercing your ears. Practicing a neutral response like "Oh, I hear you screaming. I wonder what you need" can go a long way in calming our stress response so we don't overreact and reinforce the behavior.
- **Giving the Behavior Lots of Attention:** The more attention we give something, the more likely a toddler is to do it. It's best to give attention to the behavior we *want* to see, not the behavior we do not want to see.
- **Not Teaching Skills:** We typically focus on telling a child what not to do instead of teaching them what to do. "Stop yelling! That's too loud!" Toddlers lack experience and skills and it's our job to teach them the skills they need to be successful. (And remember, it takes time to learn and practice these skills!)

If you find yourself stuck in this disempowering cycle, take heart! You're not failing, and it's never too late to make a change.

SCRIPTS FOR COMMUNICATION
Responding to Yelling

Avoid Saying: "Stop screaming!"
Try Saying: "Let's take a few deep breaths, then we'll figure this out together."

Avoid Saying: "Be quiet!"
Try Saying: "Please use a softer voice like this."

> **Avoid Saying:** "I told you to stop screaming!"
> **Try Saying:** "I can see you are frustrated. Let's figure out why. What happened?"

Breaking the Cycle

Your toddler isn't yelling to drive you crazy, even if it feels that way at times. They're yelling because they haven't yet learned how to communicate their needs effectively in a more appropriate way, or they have learned that it's an effective communication strategy. While this behavior is developmentally normal, it doesn't mean there's nothing you can do to help them transform it. This is where your guidance becomes crucial—a balance of staying calm, creating connection, setting clear limits, teaching skills, and empowering your child. The goal is to support their brain development by teaching them more effective and socially appropriate ways to express their feelings, emotions, needs, and desires.

Here's a step-by-step guide to breaking the cycle of screaming, yelling, and demands.

Step 1: Get to the Root

Start by getting curious about the behavior. What feelings, emotions, needs, or desires is your toddler trying to communicate? Is your child getting sick? Are they hungry, tired, or in pain? Sometimes we lose track of time and they suddenly have a serious case of the grumps that a simple snack can make better.

Reflect internally and voice your observations out loud to your child. *Connection is your superpower*—help your toddler feel seen and heard. Saying, "You're yelling. I wonder if you're feeling frustrated because I didn't understand what you want" acknowledges their emotions and opens the door to healthier communication.

Step 2: Don't Immediately React

When your toddler yells for a toy, snack, or your attention, the temptation to give in for a moment of peace is strong. Instead, pause. Take a deep breath. Resist the urge to comply immediately.

By waiting until your child calms down or uses a quieter voice before granting their request, you're teaching them that screaming isn't the way to get what they want.

In action, this could look like getting down on their level and saying, "I hear you want a snack. You can say, 'Snack, please,'" then pausing to give your child a chance to practice a redo.

Step 3: Teach Skills

Just like you wouldn't expect a child to solve a math problem before they've learned how, we can't expect them to wait patiently, express themselves clearly, or make independent choices without support. These are skills—just like tying shoes or counting to ten. Instead of focusing on what not to do, ask yourself: *What is my child ready to learn?* Whether it's taking turns, saying how they feel, or pouring their own water, everyday moments become powerful opportunities to build independence, communication, and impulse control—one small step at a time.

Independence Skills

- Empower your child to meet their needs independently.
- Example: If your toddler frequently demands water, set up a small pitcher and sponge on a tray for them to practice pouring. Gradually increase their autonomy by adding a water dispenser at their height.

Communication Skills

- Model simple phrases and the tone they can use, such as "Help, please" or "I need a snack," especially when they are making a demand.
- Use visual aids, like picture cards, to help them communicate their needs (e.g., a picture of a cup for water).
- Teach basic signs for key requests like "more," "help," or "thank you," especially for toddlers still developing verbal skills.

Social and Emotional Skills
- Help your toddler recognize and name their emotions. Try saying, "I wonder if you're feeling angry or frustrated. Let's talk about it."
- Role-play common scenarios during playtime, using toys or puppets to practice calm communication.
- Reinforce these skills during calm moments by modeling positive behaviors and celebrating their efforts.

Step 4: Practice Patience and Impulse Control

Toddlers are wired for instant gratification—waiting is not a skill that comes naturally. But just like muscles, patience and self-control can be strengthened over time. The trick is to teach through play, keep expectations age-appropriate, and stay consistent. When we make waiting feel doable and even fun, we help wire their brains for flexibility and resilience. It won't happen overnight, but with practice, they'll surprise you.

- Teach patience through fun games like Simon Says or Red Light, Green Light. These activities promote listening, waiting, and following instructions.
- Use a visual timer to make time tangible. Then explain to your child, "You want Mommy to read a book. When all the sand is at the bottom of the timer, I'll read it."
- Praise their efforts: "You waited patiently for your sandwich. Thank you!"

Step 5: Model the Behavior You Want to See

Your toddler is constantly observing you. Practice speaking calmly, even when you are frustrated. By modeling effective communication, you show them how to handle emotions and situations constructively.

Step 6: Support Sensory and Emotional Needs

If your child's screaming stems from sensory challenges, help them regulate with sensory strategies (discussed in chapter 12, "Getting to Know Your Toddler's Sensory System").

For emotional overwhelm, offer physical comfort and validation.

Help them find their emotional equilibrium before addressing the issue further.

Step 7: Adjust Expectations

Understand your toddler's developmental capabilities and align your expectations accordingly.

For a Younger Toddler: Focus on modeling behavior and teaching communication skills, understanding that they lack impulse control and will need plenty of practice before showing change. For example, if your toddler is yelling, you might say, "I hear you yelling, and I'm trying to understand what you want." Then point to different items and say, "I wonder if you're saying . . ." Once you figure it out, respond by teaching them more about what they are trying to communicate: "Oh, you want strawberries! You can say, 'Strawberries, please!'" This models the language, even though your toddler may not yet be able to repeat it, as comprehension develops before speech.

For an Older Toddler: Emphasize teaching impulse control and encouraging them to practice better ways of communicating. Acknowledge their effort while holding space for mistakes. For instance, if they're yelling for a snack, you might say, "I hear you yelling for a snack. I'm happy to help! Let's try asking in a better way—'Papa, I want a snack, please.'"

The cycle of screaming and demands can feel relentless, but with patience, consistency, and a bit of strategy, you can break it. By not giving in immediately, teaching alternative communication, and modeling the behavior you want to see, you empower your child to develop healthier ways of expressing their needs—and reclaim some peace and calm for yourself in the process.

FAQs

Sometimes I lose my patience and yell at my toddler. Am I teaching them to yell?

We are all human and will lose our patience from time to time. It's true that toddlers are little mirrors who reflect our words and actions back to us, and if we constantly raise our voices to get our toddlers to listen, we're teaching them that yelling is how to be heard. It's also true that you don't have to be a perfect parent to be a good parent. If you find yourself yelling daily, please know that you are not alone. You are a good parent who needs more support. Please read chapters 7, 8, and 9 for more support.

Chapter 23

RESPONDING TO WHINING

You're sitting at your kitchen table, attempting to meal plan for the next week. The room is silent except for the occasional rustle of paper or the soft sound of your pen scratching on a page. You feel calm, focused, ready to tackle the task at hand.

Now, picture that same scenario—but instead of silence, you're surrounded by the sound of whining. It's incessant, piercing, and impossible to ignore. Your concentration wavers, your patience frays, and suddenly, some simple planning feels like an insurmountable challenge. And it's not just you! Research shows that whining is more distracting and stressing to our brains and nervous systems than infant cries.[1] It's a sound that triggers a primal reaction, one that's difficult to ignore because it's rooted in the basic human need to address distress.

This serves as a powerful reminder of the impact that whining can have, not just on our nerves but also on our ability to function and respond effectively. In other words? When faced with a whiny toddler, it's no wonder you sometimes feel like you're drowning and ready to snap!

Why Toddlers Whine

For toddlers, whining is a tool. It's how they communicate their needs when they don't yet have the words to express themselves and how they attempt to assert control over their environment. Rather than viewing whining as an irritating behavior to ignore, recognize it as a signal that something in your little one's world needs attention.

Whining isn't just a random noise; it's an early form of communication. It's your toddler's way of saying, "I feel disconnected," "I feel overwhelmed," or "I have an unmet need." Sure, it can sound like nails on a chalkboard—no parent enjoys hearing it—but that irritation can sometimes cloud what's really happening. Whining is your child's SOS, a call for help.

> **TODDLER TIP**
> *Tune In to Whining*
>
> When your child whines, take it as a signal to tune in and uncover what they are trying to communicate instead of a reason to ignore them. Whining, like all behavior, is a form of communication.

In younger toddlers, whining often stems from their lack of vocabulary to articulate what they need, heightening their frustration. In older toddlers, as language skills and independence grow, whining becomes a way to test limits and exert control—because they've learned it will grab your attention. Understanding the reasons behind whining can help you respond with empathy, patience, and strategies that foster connection while maintaining limits.

Here are some of the most common reasons why toddlers whine:

- emotional or sensory overwhelm
- unmet needs
- inadequate communication skills
- feeling disconnected from you
- not feeling seen and heard
- lacking patience and impulse control
- exploring limits and boundaries

What to Do and What Not to Do When Whining Starts

When your child begins to whine, it's important to handle it in a way that doesn't reinforce the behavior and also aims to meet your child's needs within your boundaries. Here are my recommendations.

What to Do

- **Stay Calm:** Keep your voice calm and steady. Remember, you're modeling the behavior you want to see.
- **Acknowledge Your Child:** Start by using the four magic words—"I hear you saying . . ."—then insert what your child said. If you have a younger toddler who isn't speaking yet, you can say, "I wonder if you are trying to tell me . . ." then insert what you think your toddler wants. Or if you can't understand your child, you might say, "I can't understand you and I want to help."
- **Get Curious:** Get curious about what your child is trying to communicate behind their words. What's at the root of the whining? You can even do this out loud: "I wonder if there is something bothering you." "I wonder what you are trying to tell me."
- **Encourage Communication:** Model the tone of voice and word choices you want your toddler to use. If you have an older toddler, offer them a redo: "Please ask me using a calm voice like this." "Let's take a deep breath and try again." For a younger toddler, you can still model this knowing that, while they won't be able to practice a redo, they are learning from you: "Snack, please."

What to Avoid

- **Giving In:** Avoid giving in to the whining. This will only teach your child that whining works to get their needs and desires met.
- **Reacting with Frustration:** Raising your voice or showing frustration can escalate the situation, reinforce the behavior, and shatter emotional safety.

- **Ignoring Your Child:** While it's important not to reinforce whining, ignoring your child can lead to more intense behaviors as they try harder to get your attention and communicate.
- **Unrealistic Expectations:** Avoid asking your child to "use your words." They would be using their words if they could in that moment. The goal is to meet your child where they are, not demand where you wish they were.

SCRIPTS FOR COMMUNICATION
Turning Frustration into Communication

Whining isn't just noise—it's a signal. Toddlers don't whine to annoy us (even if it grates on every nerve); they whine because they're overwhelmed, under-skilled, or unsure of how to ask for what they need. Instead of shutting it down with dismissive phrases like "Stop whining," we can use those moments as opportunities to model respectful communication. With just a few small shifts in our words, we teach our children how to express big feelings in better ways, while showing them that their voice matters.

Avoid Saying	Try Saying
"Stop whining."	"I hear you saying you want to stay home."
"Use a nice/polite voice."	"Please use a talking voice like this."
"I won't help you when you talk like that."	"I'm here to help you. Let's try that again."
"Use your words."	"Let's find a word that helps you say what you want/need/feel."

When we respond with patience and intention, we don't just stop the whining—we build trust, teach communication, and show our children that they can count on us to truly listen.

Preventing Whining: Proactive Strategies

Preventing whining starts with understanding the triggers that lead to it. Often, whining occurs when a child is tired, hungry, or feeling overwhelmed. By addressing these needs proactively, you can reduce the likelihood of whining before it even starts. Here are some strategies to help prevent whining:

- **Establish Routines:** Consistent routines create a sense of predictability and can help your child feel secure and ensure their needs are met.
- **Teach and Model Skills:** Help your child build their vocabulary and express their needs with words and baby sign language. Role-playing different scenarios can be a fun way to practice.
- **Provide Choices:** Giving your child choices throughout the day can help them feel more in control and make them less likely to whine.
- **Offer Positive Reinforcement:** When your child communicates effectively without whining, acknowledge them: "Thanks for asking me in a calm voice." Positive reinforcement encourages the behavior you want to see.

The next time that high-pitched sound pierces the air, you'll be ready—not just to stop it but to understand it and guide your child to a better way of communicating.

Remember: There is not just one "right" way to respond. Just like all behavior, whining is about what's beneath the surface: the feelings, emotions, needs, and desires at the root of the behavior. Curiosity will help you create connection and uncover what is happening.

RESPONDING TO WHINING WITH CONNECTION AND BOUNDARIES

Scenario

Your child is whining for a cookie and it's almost time for dinner.

Option 1: Give a Sense of Control

"I hear you saying you want a cookie, and I can't give it to you right now. It's almost dinnertime. Do you want to keep playing for ten more minutes or help set the table?"

Option 2: Meet the Need Within Your Boundaries

"I wonder if you are feeling hungry. It's almost time for dinner. Would you like a piece of the cookie or a piece of a banana?"

Option 3: Set a Limit If Needed

"I hear you saying you want a cookie. You can have one with dinner." If your child cries, say: "It's hard to wait. You want it right now."

Option 4: Model Positive Behavior

"I wonder if you are feeling hungry. Would you like something to eat? Okay. When you want something to eat, you can ask like this: 'Snack, please.'"

FAQs

Is it normal for my toddler to whine all the time?

Whining is a completely normal and developmentally appropriate behavior for toddlers. It's often their go-to way of expressing frustration, fatigue, or unmet needs because they're still learning more effective communication skills. However, whining can unintentionally become a habit if it consistently helps a child get what they want. To avoid reinforcing the behavior, practice consistently upholding the limits you set and avoid appeasing your child by giving in to their whining. Additionally, if your child is struggling emotionally or having sensory challenges, they may use whining to try to communicate this.

Why is my child's whining so triggering?

Whining can be incredibly triggering for many parents, and the reasons often run deeper than the surface frustration. For some, it stirs up memories of being shamed or dismissed as a child for expressing similar emotions, leading them to view whining as inherently "bad" behavior. Others may feel responsible for their child's happiness and internalize the whining as a personal failure: *If my child is whining, I must be doing something wrong.* Additionally, whining can amplify feelings of being out of control, triggering stress and overwhelm. The key is recognizing that your reaction isn't just about the whining—it's often tied to underlying beliefs, past experiences, or the natural challenges of parenting. Taking a moment to pause, breathe, and remind yourself that this phase is normal can help you respond with more calm and compassion.

Should I ignore whining?

No, ignoring whining isn't the solution. While outdated parenting advice often suggests ignoring whining to "teach a lesson," this approach overlooks the fact that whining is your child's attempt to communicate their feelings, emotions, and needs. Young children don't need to be ignored. Instead, focus on *connection*: Validate their feelings, set clear limits, and guide them toward better communication.

Chapter 24

ADDRESSING HURTFUL WORDS

Out of nowhere, your sweet little one hits you with a sharp "You're mean!" Ouch. It stings, doesn't it? It's hard not to take it personally when those big, innocent eyes glare up at you and deliver words that cut deep. Your adult brain, wired to analyze and interpret, takes those words at face value. Suddenly, your heart is in your throat, and the sting triggers feelings of sadness, anger, or even self-doubt. Your mind might instantly snap to, "How dare you be so disrespectful!"

But here's the truth: Your toddler isn't being disrespectful, nor are they out to hurt you. Starting around ages three to four, toddlers begin experimenting with using words to convey their emotions. The bigger the emotions, the stronger the words they'll use to try to match how they feel.

This behavior is impulsive, emotionally driven, and totally developmentally appropriate. It's messy, imperfect, and part of the process of learning to express themselves. Those hurtful words? They're not personal attacks—they're the verbal equivalent of flailing arms when your child feels overwhelmed by big emotions. What used to be physical outbursts like kicking, screaming, or biting are now shifting to verbal expressions.

When your toddler blurts out "You're mean!" or "I don't like you!" what they're really saying is, "I'm upset, and I don't know how to deal with it!" They're frustrated, scared, or disappointed and reaching for the most powerful words they know to communicate those feelings and get the message across.

Why Guilt Doesn't Work

It's tempting to respond with frustration or guilt-inducing statements like "You're hurting Daddy's feelings" or "That makes me sad when you say that." But guilt isn't an effective way to change behavior. In fact, it can create fear—fear of losing your love and acceptance, which is every child's deepest concern. Also, it can be scary for a child to have power over us. When that fear is triggered, their behavior often gets worse, not better.

Making your child responsible for your emotions isn't just ineffective—it's a form of manipulation. Over time, it teaches kids to prioritize others' feelings over their own, setting them up for unhealthy dynamics like people-pleasing and resentment. Instead of shaming children into listening, follow these three steps to respond with empathy and intention:

1. **Stay Neutral:** Take a deep breath and put on your poker face. Remind yourself that this is not an emergency. Calm yourself first so you can respond intentionally, not react emotionally or take it personally.
2. **Translate the Message:** Hurtful words often signal that your child is struggling to express big emotions. Instead of taking the words at face value, get curious and reflect their feelings back:
    - "It's disappointing that screen time is over."
    - "I wonder if you're feeling frustrated. Can we talk about it?"
3. **Set Limits and Teach Skills:** Empathy doesn't mean letting hurtful behavior slide. You can validate their feelings while calmly setting boundaries:
    - "It's frustrating to be told no when you want something. Saying 'I don't like you' is hurtful. You can say 'I'm mad' when you feel this way."

What your toddler needs most in these moments is to feel seen and understood. You can achieve this by translating the message to get to the root of the words. By staying calm, creating connection, and teaching better ways to communicate big feelings verbally, you help them navigate their feelings in a healthy way. Over time, this teaches them how to express themself in a more acceptable way while strengthening the trust between you.

ADDRESSING HURTFUL WORDS

So instead of hearing "I don't like you anymore!" listen for the emotion or need behind the words: "I feel hurt," "I'm scared," or "I'm disappointed." Focusing on the emotion, not the words, shifts the dynamic from conflict to connection and helps your toddler learn the skills they need to communicate more effectively in the future.

SCRIPTS FOR COMMUNICATION
Responding to "Go Away!"

Toddlers say "go away" because they are feeling upset and don't know how to communicate "I'm angry" or "I'm disappointed" when they are experiencing those big emotions. They may also say it to test your unconditional love or to satisfy their question of *Will Mom or Dad still love me even when I feel out of control?*

The best thing to do is approach your toddler with patience and aim for connection, so you can share your calm and help them meet the limit while supporting their big emotions.

Avoid	Try
Reacting to the Behavior: "That's not a nice thing to say. Fine. I'm going to leave then."	Respecting the Boundary: "I hear you saying 'go away.' It seems like you want some space. I'll move back here."
Making Your Toddler Responsible for Your Emotions: "You are making me so sad."	Giving Reassurance: "I hear you. That is NOT what you wanted to happen!"
Taking It Personally: "Why are you being so rude and hurtful?"	Being Honest: "I want to help you and I'm not sure how."
Addressing the Surface Behavior First: "Stop saying that right now!"	Addressing the Root of the Behavior First: "I wonder if you're upset. What's going on?"

Swear Words

Hearing your child's first words is one of the most exciting milestones of parenting little ones. Yet hearing your child's first *swear* word can be downright shocking and terrifying. It's like a record screeching to a halt—your heart skips a beat, and all the oxygen seems to leave the room. Did they just say . . . what I think they said? The shock, the horror, the immediate panic—how do you even begin to address this?

First, take a deep breath. Remember, your child is experimenting. They've heard a new word, maybe from you, maybe from that one episode of your favorite show that you thought they weren't paying attention to, and now they're testing it out. They might not fully understand what it means, but they do understand that it got a big reaction from you, and that's intriguing.

The key to handling your toddler's experimentation with swear words? Don't make a big deal out of it. Toddlers are little scientists—they're constantly testing the waters to see what gets a reaction. If you gasp, laugh, or otherwise react strongly, you're fueling their curiosity and unintentionally reinforcing the behavior. Instead, try to stay calm, act like nothing happened, and redirect their attention elsewhere.

But what if they keep saying the word, hoping to get that same reaction from you? This is where you get curious. Ask yourself, *What is my child really trying to communicate? Are they frustrated? Testing boundaries? Seeking attention?* By getting to the root of the behavior, you can address the underlying need rather than just the surface-level action. If the behavior continues, acknowledge your child's need to be seen and heard in a calm and validating way. Here are a few examples of calm, validating responses to swearing:

- "It seems like you really want us to know you can say ____."
- "I wonder if you're curious about how we'll react when you say ____."
- "Are you trying to get my attention by saying this word?"

After you've chosen one of these responses, you can redirect: "Let's find another word to say instead."

This approach helps your child feel understood while gently guiding them toward more appropriate ways to communicate.

Tools and Strategies for Addressing Hurtful and Swear Words

- **Avoid Big Reactions:** Gasping, laughing, or getting upset shows your toddler how much power they have over your emotions and reactions, which can reinforce the behavior. Instead, aim to stay as neutral as possible, almost as if nothing happened. While they may not fully understand the word or action, they quickly learn that if it grabs your attention, it gives them power. This triggers their natural developmental drive to test boundaries, assert independence, and seek connection, leading them to repeat the behavior.
- **Ignore the Behavior:** If your toddler is swearing just to see your reaction, don't give them the satisfaction. Ignore it, and it'll lose its appeal. Ignoring the behavior doesn't mean ignoring the child. This means you can still create connection or redirect.
- **Connect and Redirect:** Sometimes all your toddler needs is a little redirection. If they're swearing or saying hurtful things, redirect their attention to something else. "Hey, let's go build a tower with those blocks!"
- **Set Limits (as Needed):** If the behavior continues you can set a limit in a clear, matter-of-fact way. "This word is off-limits."
- **Translate the Words:** If your toddler says a swear word when they drop something, translate it by narrating what happened: "You dropped your banana. I wonder if you are feeling frustrated."
- **Give Them Words:** Teach your toddler the words they need to express themself. "When you feel this way, you can say, 'I'm frustrated.'" Notice that I didn't mention the swear word. I'm focusing on the behavior I want to see instead of the behavior I don't want to see.
- **Model the Behavior You Want to See:** If you use positive language and express your emotions in healthy ways, they'll follow

your lead. When you're frustrated, instead of swearing, say, "I'm feeling really frustrated right now." Show them how to handle big feelings constructively.

- **Monitor Media Consumption:** Be mindful of what your toddler is exposed to. They're absorbing more than you might realize, whether it's TV shows, music, or conversations around them. Keep their environment as positive and age-appropriate as possible.

As always, you're not expected to use every strategy. Trust that you know your child best and can choose what works for you both. When trying out new approaches, stick with them consistently for a couple of weeks before evaluating what's effective, what isn't, and how you might adjust your approach.

The next time your toddler throws a hurtful word your way, or when that dreaded swear word pops out, take a deep breath. Translate the message, teach the skills, and know that you're guiding them through one of the most important lessons of all: how to navigate their big, beautiful, and sometimes overwhelming world of emotions.

FAQs

My toddler is using potty talk. How do I make it stop?

There are a few different ways to respond, but the most important thing is to stay completely neutral—like it doesn't faze you at all. Avoid reacting or over-engaging. Most of the time, the behavior will fade on its own.

If it doesn't, you can respond in a literal and matter-of-fact way: "I hear you saying 'pee-pee caca.' Do you need to go to the bathroom?" If the answer is no, simply move on.

Another approach is to meet your child's need to express themself while maintaining boundaries: "I hear you saying 'poo-poo butt.' You can say those words in the bathroom or in your room." Then calmly redirect them to the appropriate space.

Be mindful, though—if you're not careful, it's easy to get stuck in a power struggle. Stay consistent, clear, and composed to guide them without escalating the situation.

My child called me *stupid*. What should I do?

The most important thing here is to rise above the behavior and not take it personally. It can be tempting to immediately punish your child for being "disrespectful," but doing so can unintentionally communicate "You don't have my unconditional love when you act this way." This message can backfire, worsening the behavior as your child feels less connected to their emotional anchor. Remember, this is *not* disrespectful behavior. It's communication.

Instead, focus on creating emotional safety. Start by interpreting the behavior: "I wonder if you are feeling upset about not going to the park—so upset that you said, 'You're stupid' to me." Then guide your child toward a healthier form of self-expression. You might even encourage a redo to reinforce the skill.

Once your child is calm, have a conversation about how powerful certain words can be and how to repair relationships after using them. (For more on repairing relationships, see chapter 8, "Becoming a Safe Parent.") By modeling connection, understanding, and accountability, you help your child learn to navigate big emotions while preserving the trust between you.

Chapter 25

COPING WITH PARENTAL PREFERENCE

Part of the process of your toddler becoming their own person is discovering and communicating their preferences. From the color of their cup to the spot where they want to sit at the dinner table, their choices can be as firm as they are fleeting. But what about when it comes to parental preference—the moment your little one decides they want nothing but one parent all day, every day?

Parental preference is one of those developmental phases that often catches parents off guard, leaving one parent feeling like the rock star while the other feels like a backup singer—needed, but not the headliner.

Whether you're the favored parent basking in the glow of toddler adoration, or the less preferred parent navigating the sting of rejection, it's important to remember that this, too, shall pass. It's developmentally driven, it's not personal, and yes, there are ways to navigate this phase with grace, unity, and maybe even a bit of humor.

The *Why* Behind Parental Preference

Let's clear something up: Parental preference does not mean that one parent is better than the other. It doesn't mean your child loves one parent more. I know this is how it can *feel* in the moment, but remember: Feelings aren't facts. *Feelings are reactions to the facts.*

Example of a Feeling vs. a Fact
Feeling: My child doesn't love me.
Fact: My child wanted Daddy to do bath time again.

What it does mean is that your toddler is knee-deep in a phase where they're figuring out who they are, what they want, and how much power they have over their world. So why does this happen? Here's a glimpse into the toddler mind:

- **Showing Independence:** Your toddler is starting to see themself as a separate individual, and one way they assert that independence is by making choices—often loudly and with conviction. Choosing one parent over the other is just another way of saying, "I'm my own person, and I get to decide!"
- **Experimenting and Exploring:** Toddlers are natural experimenters. They want to know how the world works, including how people react to their demands. Parental preference is often a way for them to test boundaries, see how far they can push, and explore the dynamics of power in relationships.
- **Routine Associations:** When one parent regularly handles a specific task or routine, the child may associate that parent with comfort and predictability. This familiarity can create a strong attachment, making the other parent seem less connected to that routine. However, sometimes the opposite can also happen—especially during separation-anxiety phases—when the less present parent becomes the preferred one because their limited availability feels special or more valuable.
- **Separation Anxiety:** When your toddler clings to one parent, it's often a reflection of their anxiety about separation. They might feel like they need to protect their time with the preferred parent, seeing the other parent as a potential threat to that connection.

The good news? This phase is not inherently bad and is temporary. And while it can be tough on everyone involved, it's also a sign that your child feels secure enough in your love to push boundaries and explore these dynamics.

The Challenges of Being the Preferred Parent

Being the preferred parent might sound like a dream come true, but it comes with its own set of challenges. When you're the favored one, you might feel a mix of pride, exhaustion, and even guilt. After all, it's hard to say no when your toddler wants you—whether it's at bedtime, during a meltdown, or when they're hurt.

Here's what to keep in mind if you find yourself in the preferred-parent role:

- **Resist the Urge to "Rescue":** It's hard to watch your toddler struggle with their feelings, especially when they're asking for you. But swooping in to rescue them from the non-preferred parent can reinforce the idea that the other parent can't handle things. Set clear limits on when and how you will step in and then follow through.
- **Take Care of Yourself:** It's easy to lose yourself in your child's needs when you're the preferred parent. Make sure you're taking time for self-care, even if it means stepping away and letting the other parent take the reins.

The Challenges of Being the Non-Preferred Parent

Now, let's talk about what it's like to be the non-preferred parent. It's tough. It stings. And it can leave you questioning your role in your child's life. But being the non-preferred parent isn't a reflection of your worth or your ability to connect with your child. It's just a phase—and one that can be navigated with patience, empathy, and a little bit of strategy. If you're feeling the sting of being less preferred, here's what you can do:

- **Don't Take It Personally:** This is easier said than done, but it's crucial. Remember that your toddler's preference is developmentally driven—it's not about you. They're exploring their independence, testing boundaries, and navigating their feelings of attachment and separation.
- **Validate Your Child's Feelings:** When your toddler asks for the other parent, it's easy to feel rejected. But instead of reacting defensively, try to validate their feelings. Acknowledge their desire for the preferred parent. This helps create a sense of connection and shows them that you're on their team.
- **Avoid Power Struggles:** It's easy to fall into a power struggle when your toddler demands the other parent. But instead of forcing the issue, try to remain calm and patient. Acknowledge their feelings but hold firm to the boundaries you've set. Remember, it's not about winning—it's about supporting your child's emotional needs.

Strategies for Navigating Parental Preference as a Team

When it comes to parental preference, the most important thing you and your partner can do is work together as a team. Toddlers are experts at detecting inconsistencies, and if they sense a divide between you, they'll use it strategically to get their needs met—often without even realizing it. Here are my top tips for how to navigate this phase together, without letting it drive a wedge between you:

1. **Create a Game Plan:** Sit down with your partner and discuss how you'll handle situations where parental preference usually happens. Decide on specific strategies you'll use, such as who will handle bedtime or how you'll respond to demands for the

preferred parent. The more prepared you are, the less likely you are to get caught off guard.

2. **Stay Connected with Each Other:** Parental preference can be tough on your relationship, so make sure you're staying connected with your partner. Regularly check in with each other about how you're feeling and offer support when needed. Remember, you're in this together.

3. **Avoid Competing for Your Child's Affection:** It's natural to want to be the "favorite" parent, but competing for your child's affection can create tension and insecurity. Instead, focus on supporting each other and building a strong, united front. Your child needs to see that both parents are equally capable and equally important.

4. **Start Slowly and Build the Relationship:** If your child is strongly attached to one parent, it's important to start slowly and build the relationship with the non-preferred parent over time in a non-threatening way. The preferred parent can begin by doing more activities outside the home, allowing the non-preferred parent to spend more one-on-one time with the child doing activities they love. Gradually, the child will start to feel more comfortable with the non-preferred parent.

5. **Incorporate the Non-Preferred Parent into Routine Activities:** Instead of making a complete handoff, try incorporating the non-preferred parent into routine activities in a gentle way. For example, if your child wants the preferred parent to read them a bedtime story, have the non-preferred parent join in and take turns. Or if your child wants the preferred parent to give the bath, have both parents give the bath. Then, once your child accepts that, have the preferred parent start stepping away for a short moment. Over time, extend how long the preferred parent is stepping away.

6. **Give Your Child a Sense of Control:** Toddlers love to feel in control, so try giving your child some choices within the boundaries you've set. For example, you can ask your child to choose which parent reads the bedtime story first or what activity they'd like to do with the non-preferred parent.

7. **Reflect and Adjust as Needed:** As you navigate this phase, take time to reflect on what's working and what's not. If something isn't working, don't be afraid to adjust your approach. The goal is to create a supportive environment where your child feels secure with both parents.
8. **Focus on Connection, Not Perfection:** Building a relationship with your child takes time, especially if they have a strong preference for the other parent. Focus on creating small moments of connection rather than striving for perfection. Over time, these small moments will add up and strengthen your bond.

Again, parental preference is a phase, and like all phases, it will pass. Be patient with yourself, your partner, and your child as you navigate this period. The more you can remain calm, consistent, and supportive, the quicker the phase will likely pass.

FAQs

How long does parental preference last?

Parental preference can last anywhere from a few days to several months—or even longer. Every child is different, and their preferences can shift unpredictably. It's also common for preferences to flip-flop between parents and specific activities. For example, your child might insist for months that only one parent put them to bed, then suddenly switch and demand the other parent instead. These changes are a normal part of toddler development as they explore independence, attachment, and control in their environment.

How should we deal with parental preference at bedtime?

Start by deciding what works within your family's boundaries. If it's manageable for one parent to consistently handle bedtime, you might agree to stick with that routine. However, if you want both parents involved, create a consistent schedule that rotates responsibility. For example, alternate nights or split bedtime duties, such as one parent managing bath time while the other handles story time. When you hear "I want Daddy!" try saying, "I hear you want Daddy. You love being with him. We both love you so much. Tonight is my turn to put you to bed. Daddy will put you to bed tomorrow night." Remember, only set limits you are willing to follow through on.

Chapter 26

NAVIGATING SCREEN TIME CONFIDENTLY

When it comes to toddlers and screen time, I know the struggle is real. If you've ever handed your toddler a tablet just to get five minutes of peace, you're not alone. And let's be honest, the guilt probably settled in right after. But let's shake off that guilt, shall we? This isn't about finger-pointing or playing the blame game. We're here to figure out how to navigate this digital jungle with our sanity intact and our toddlers thriving.

Screens often feel like our lifeline—our break, our ace up the sleeve in navigating the chaos of daily life. The truth is this is the first generation growing up with screens woven so deeply into every aspect of our lives. While a wealth of research exists on screen time, there's still so much more to uncover. The goal is to empower you to make informed decisions that suit your unique family—decisions about how screens do or don't play a role in your life so you can create positive habits around them.

How Screens Impact the Brain

To understand why screen time can be such a double-edged sword, we need to take another peek inside your toddler's brain. Remember that fireworks show of neural connections? Toddlerhood is a sensitive period for brain development, and screens (especially excessive use of them) can throw a wrench into that process. The bright colors, rapid pace, and constant visual and cognitive stimulation in shows and apps can overwhelm the sensory system, creating **sensory overload**. This overload can lead to a state of **hyperarousal**, keeping your child's brain on high alert when it should be winding down.

The result? The brain's reward system being hijacked and rewired. The bright lights and fast action trigger the release of dopamine, the brain's feel-good chemical. Dopamine is tied to pleasure, attention, and even motor activity, but it's also involved in addiction. Once that dopamine starts flowing, your toddler is hooked, craving more quick hits of pleasure.

Over time, this repeated stimulation can rewire the brain. Children can begin to crave screen time and the dopamine hit that comes with it rather than the slower, steadier work of unstructured play and building emotional regulation. Chronic sensory overload can lead to **chronic stress**, causing blood flow to shift away from the frontal lobe—the area responsible for decision-making and emotional regulation—and toward more primitive areas of the brain. This can make toddlers more reactive, more defensive, and less empathetic. And the effects don't stop there. The cumulative impact of repeated screen overexposure can leave their inner world feeling chaotic, leading to struggles with paying attention, acting out, and desperately seeking to control the world around them.

The kicker? These effects are **synergistic** and **cumulative**, so you might not notice them right away. It's easy to miss that screen time is the root cause of a more chaotic, overstimulated brain. But as the foundations of attention, empathy, and emotional resilience are laid, relying on screens is like trying to build a house on quicksand—it's only a matter of time before cracks begin to show.

Deciding on How Much and When to Give Screen Time

When deciding whether and how much screen time to allow your child, there are many factors to consider. Screen time has positive and negative aspects—it's about creating healthy habits within your family. Let's dive into some of the potential risks and benefits, backed by research.

Potential Risks

When overused or unregulated, screen time can have the following significant negative effects on a child's development:

- **Disrupted Sleep and Obesity Risk:** Research has found that excessive screen use (more than an hour per day for toddlers) correlates with shorter sleep duration and increased obesity risk due to disrupted sleep rhythms and sedentary behavior.[1]
- **More Meltdowns and Power Struggles:** Excessive screen time is linked to heightened emotional dysregulation, leading to more frequent meltdowns and power struggles, especially when screens are used before bedtime.[2]
- **Increased Reactivity:** Reliance on mobile devices for emotional regulation in children aged three to five is associated with decreased executive functioning and heightened emotional reactivity over time.[3]
- **Disrupted Attention Span:** Overuse of screens, particularly depending on content type and duration, may hinder a child's ability to sustain focus.[4]
- **Delayed Language Development:** Excessive unsupervised television viewing in children under two years old is linked to delayed language development, while reading aloud to toddlers is significantly more beneficial.[5]
- **Decreased Emotional Well-Being:** Studies show that beyond one hour of daily screen use, children experience lower well-being, including reduced curiosity, self-control, and emotional stability, and increased distractibility.[6]

Potential Positives

When used in moderation and with high-quality content, screen time can also offer the following benefits:

- **Family Bonding:** Watching educational shows or movies together can be a shared family activity that fosters connection.
- **Parental Relief:** Screens can provide parents with a much-needed break, creating opportunities for self-care or focused attention on other tasks.
- **Educational Opportunities:** High-quality children's programming, especially when co-viewed with parents, can support cognitive development, language skills, and digital literacy. For example, one study found that children aged three to five who watched *Sesame Street* had larger vocabularies in high school compared to children who watched other shows or no television at all.[7]

The key is to create mindful screen habits tailored to your child's temperament, needs, and developmental stage plus your family's values while avoiding excessive screen time. If you do decide to offer your child screen time, opt for age-appropriate, high-quality content, set clear boundaries, and, whenever possible, engage with your child during screen time to make it a meaningful experience. One important question to ask yourself before giving screen time is *What would my child be doing if they weren't having screen time? What activity or opportunity is this taking them away from?* It's vital to balance screens with activities like reading, outdoor play, and creative exploration to build a well-rounded foundation for your child's growth.

SCREEN TIME RECOMMENDATIONS FROM THE AMERICAN ACADEMY OF ADOLESCENT AND CHILD PSYCHIATRY

- Until eighteen months of age, screen time should be limited to video chatting with the help of an adult.
- Between eighteen and twenty-four months, "screen time should be limited to watching educational programming with a caregiver."

- For children ages two to five, noneducational screen time should not exceed one hour per weekday and three hours on the weekend days.
- For children age six and older, "encourage healthy habits and limit activities that include screens."[8]

When to Reduce Screen Time

Every child handles screen time differently, but excessive use can lead to chronic overstimulation, creating an unhealthy relationship with screens—especially for children already experiencing behavioral or emotional challenges. If your child has a hard time letting go of screens, it's an early warning sign to cut back.

So how do you know when screen time is doing more harm than good? Pay attention to your child's behavior. The following are signs that it's time to reduce screen time:

- asking about screens constantly
- struggling significantly when screen time ends
- relying on screens to get through basic activities like eating, car rides, and dressing
- losing interest in playing or going outside
- showing signs of overstimulation, such as difficulty sleeping, irritability, or frequent, intense tantrums

If you suspect screen time is negatively affecting your child, try a four-week screen-free reset. This allows the brain to recalibrate and gives you insight into how screens might be impacting your child. During this time, watch for changes in behavior such as improved mood, greater engagement, more regulation, and fewer tantrums. I've had several clients do this and they have been positively shocked by the results. It's not magic—it's the brain rediscovering balance.

Steps to Go Screen-Free for Four Weeks

1. **Set the Limit:** Be clear and direct by saying, "We are taking a break from screen time."
2. **Validate Emotions:** Acknowledge your child's feelings about the change and provide emotional support. "You really want to watch *Bluey*, and you can't. I'm here to help."
3. **Follow Through:** Stay consistent. Honor the limit and hold firm to the screen-free period even if your child protests.
4. **Observe and Track Changes:** Keep notes on shifts in behavior, mood, and interactions.

After a reset, you may notice several positive changes in your toddler. Their play might become more creative and focused, and their overall attitude happier and more agreeable with less whining. You might also see an increase in verbal communication, more smiles and laughter, and better listening and connection between you. Additionally, tantrums may become shorter and less frequent, making those challenging moments easier to navigate.

Then, you can decide how and when to reintroduce screens in a way that supports a healthier relationship or to continue without screens. Use this opportunity to establish new limits, prioritize quality content, and involve your child in creating balanced screen habits.

TODDLER TIP
What to Do When It's Hard to End Screen Time

When it's tough to turn off the screen and transition your toddler to another activity, try getting down to their level and using these four magic words: *You wish you could.*

For example: "You wish you could watch *Bluey* all day long. It's one of your favorites—you just love watching it!"

> Then pause and let your child respond. This simple phrase helps your toddler feel seen, heard, and understood. Acknowledging their feelings without jumping straight into "Screen time is over!" can ease the transition and create a moment of connection before moving on.
>
> Also, try giving your child a sense of control: "Do you want to turn it off or have Daddy do it?" If they scream no, follow through: "You don't want to turn it off, so I will this time." Don't be afraid if your child has big emotions after. Stay steady and calm.

Choosing Developmentally Appropriate Content

If you're going to let your little one dive into screen time, choosing the right content can make a huge difference. The trick is to choose high-quality, age-appropriate content that won't leave their brain feeling like it just sprinted a marathon.

What to Look for in a Show or App

When selecting a show or app, consider these criteria:

- **Low Stimulation:** Content that is calm and avoids sensory overload. Look for content with these features:
    - slow pacing and very few screen transitions
    - less intense or more muted colors
    - relaxing or soothing music
    - characters that talk calmly instead of yelling
    - few to no sound effects
- **Developmentally Appropriate:** Content that matches your child's age and stage of development. Keep in mind, just because something is animated doesn't mean it's appropriate for toddlers. Even beloved classics, like Disney movies, can be overwhelming or scary.

Young children often cannot distinguish between reality and fantasy, and what seems funny to adults can be frightening to a child.

- **Models Positive Behavior:** Shows that demonstrate kindness, cooperation, problem-solving, and other values that align with your family's.
- **Pre-Watched or Co-Watched by an Adult:** Content that has been vetted to ensure it aligns with your values. Whenever you can, preview a show or movie in advance or watch it together with your child. This lets you monitor the content, observe how your child reacts, and step in to turn it off if needed.
- **No Levels or Stages:** Apps or games that do not encourage advancing by "winning," which can overstimulate and create frustration.

By being intentional about screen time, you can help ensure it remains a positive, balanced part of your child's day if you choose it for your family.

> For a downloadable list of my favorite shows and apps, as well as my favorite audio players and screen time alternatives, visit transformingtoddlerhood.com/bookresources.

TODDLER TIP
Finding Screen Time Alternatives

Prepare the environment to support you and your child in reducing screen time with these tips:

- Block five minutes before bed to set up an activity for first thing in the morning.
- Focus on play that engages more than one sense (think sensory bins).

- Get outside regardless of the weather (unless it's extreme).
- Pare down toys and rotate them every other week.
- Get your child involved in household tasks.
- Utilize audio stories and podcasts for kids.

Creating Positive Habits with Screens

Finally, let's look at the bigger picture. Screens aren't going anywhere. They're a part of our lives and society. So it's important to focus on creating a positive relationship with screens—for our children and for ourselves. Your child is always learning from you, even when it comes to how you use screens. When you model mindful screen habits and a balanced approach, they're more likely to follow your lead.

TODDLER TIP
Why Your Screen Consumption Matters

Research shows that parents who frequently use mobile devices around their children tend to display lower emotional intelligence, engage less with their kids, and respond more harshly to attention-seeking behaviors. Their children, in turn, are more likely to develop emotional and behavioral problems and may escalate their behavior in an effort to regain their parents' attention.[9]

I want to be clear that if you use your phone in front of your child, you are *not* a bad parent. This is an invitation to reexamine your screen use and be more mindful of when you check social media, respond to texts, and shop online.

Here are a few things you can try:

> - **Keep Your Phone on Silent:** Set specific phone-free hours to stay fully present.
> - **Leave Your Phone in a Basket:** During playtime, place your phone out of sight to avoid the temptation to check it. Another option is to put it in airplane mode if you want it nearby to take photos and videos.
> - **Institute a "No Phones at the Table" Rule:** Make mealtimes screen-free to encourage conversation and connection.

Ready to make a shift? Here's how to get started.

Step 1: Establish Your Family's Screen Time Values

First things first—what does your ideal relationship with screens look like? Picture your family six months to a year from now. What habits do you see? How do screens fit into your life? This isn't about perfection; it's about creating a vision that feels right for your family, whether that's more screen-free meals or dedicated downtime without digital distractions. Start by establishing your family's screen time values. What kind of relationship with technology do you want to model for your kids?

Step 2: Take Stock of Your Current Screen Time Landscape

Now, let's do a little self-reflection. What role are screens playing in your family's life right now? Be honest. Are you scrolling through your phone while playing with your child? Is the TV a constant companion during dinner? What patterns do you notice in your child's media habits, your own, and your family's as a whole? This isn't about judgment—it's about awareness. You can't change what you're not aware of.

Step 3: Make One Meaningful Change

Change doesn't have to be monumental to be effective. Think about one small adjustment you can make to move closer to that vision you created. Maybe it's as simple as setting a no-phones rule during family meals, or perhaps it's turning off the TV an hour before bedtime. Choose one change for your child, one for your family, and one for yourself. Start small, and let the ripple effect take care of the rest.

Creating positive screen time habits isn't about laying down the law with strict rules. It's about taking thoughtful, intentional steps that lead to a more balanced, empowered relationship with screens for everyone. Little by little, these small shifts can create a big difference in the long run.

Remember: You're the expert on your family. And with a little intention, a little planning, and a lot of love, you can create a screen time routine that supports your child's development and strengthens your family bond.

TODDLER TIP
Create Predictability

If you choose to give screen time on a regular basis, instead of using screen time reactively, create a predictable time each day to watch. This will increase your toddler's sense of security and reduce screen time tantrums and power struggles.

FAQs

What type of screen time is best?

There are generally two types of screen time: passive screen time (like watching a show) and interactive screen time (like playing a game on a tablet). Both can have addictive qualities. Choose shows and apps that are developmentally appropriate and have fewer addictive qualities.

Is video chatting considered screen time?

Yes—however, it's usually considered an exception for young children. Research shows that children can learn from video chatting and are more likely to benefit from it compared to noninteractive screen time, like watching TV shows or movies. Studies indicate that children as young as seventeen months can pick up language, movements, and patterns through interactive and responsive video chats.[10]

Do educational apps help my child learn?

Research shows that while children can learn certain skills from apps and screens, it's unclear whether they can effectively transfer those skills to real-world experiences. Studies also indicate that kids learn more deeply and retain information better when engaging with adults, either through direct interaction or guided learning, rather than relying solely on apps.[11]

I watched a lot of TV as a kid and I turned out fine. So what's the big deal?

Taking a one-size-fits-all approach to screen time is not useful, as the impact of screens is different for each unique child based on their sensory needs, temperament, and personality. Many of the shows for children today are specifically designed to hold their attention, resulting in more addictive qualities than shows from twenty to thirty years ago.

What type of screen is best for children?

When it comes to screen time for children, not all screens are created equal. Here's a ranking from most to least favorable:

1. **TV:** TVs are the least interactive but generally the safest option for young children. The larger screen reduces eye strain, and family viewing encourages shared experiences and discussions.
2. **Tablet:** Tablets are more interactive but safer when placed on a table rather than held. This helps maintain better posture, reduces eye strain, and minimizes accidental navigation to inappropriate content.
3. **Phone:** Phones are the least favorable due to their small screens, which can cause more eye strain. They also present more opportunities for kids to accidentally navigate to inappropriate content,

making parental supervision crucial. Phones are highly interactive but less secure for young users.

By understanding the strengths and limitations of each type of screen, you can make more informed choices about how your child engages with digital content.

Chapter 27

DISARMING POWER STRUGGLES

Ever wake up dreading the daylong tug-of-war with your toddler? It's as if you can already feel the tension in every little transition ahead: getting them dressed, convincing them to eat dinner, or buckling them into their car seat. These tasks, which seem straightforward, suddenly become monumental points of contention, leaving you drained before the day even begins.

Your toddler isn't acting out to make your life harder—they're wired to seek control. It's part of their developmental job. Toddlerhood is when they begin to realize they're separate from you and start building their sense of self. So when they dig in their heels or push back, they're not being "bad" or "difficult"—they're doing exactly what they're supposed to be doing. Their resistance is less about defiance and more about figuring out who they are in a world where so much is outside of their control.

It's not a coincidence that most powers struggles show up around bodily autonomy (sleeping, pottying, eating, getting dressed, or brushing their teeth), where they are in control of their body, and transitions (getting into a car seat, leaving the house, or cleaning up toys), where they lack control and desperately want it.

But what if I told you there was a way to shift the dynamic entirely?

A way to meet your toddler's need for independence without falling into an endless cycle of power struggles? It's possible—and it starts with reframing how you see those challenging moments.

The Shift: From Winning to Connecting

At the heart of every power struggle is a battle of wills—yours versus your toddler's. If you find yourself locked in a standoff, it's because both of you are fighting to win.

Think back to the last few power struggles you had—what were you focused on? Chances are, it was "winning." Power struggles trigger our stress response, hijacking our rational minds and launching us into survival mode. In that state, winning feels like the only option—because on a primal level, winning means surviving.

The catch? When you're laser-focused on winning, you're likely losing sight of your bigger parenting goals—teaching, guiding, and connecting. The key to breaking this cycle is recognizing that while your toddler's pushback is developmentally appropriate, your response has the power to reshape the entire interaction.

Because young children have immature brains, we can't expect them to have enough self-control at this age to disengage from a power struggle. That's *our* job. This does not mean you give up, give in, or let your child take charge and do whatever they want. The goal is to disengage without becoming permissive by using positive, respectful, developmentally appropriate tools.

Start by reframing how you see those challenging moments. Consider how the following myths could be transformed with an emphasis on connection:

- **Myth #1:** "I have to pick and choose my battles with my child."
- **Reframe:** You and your child are on the same team. There is no need to battle them.

- **Myth #2:** "It's my job to control my child."
- **Reframe:** It's your job to control yourself and influence your child while supporting their development of self-control.

These myths fuel power struggles because they're rooted in the belief that control is the goal. But control is an illusion! You can't force another human being—especially a toddler—to do anything, whether it's sleeping, eating, going to the bathroom, apologizing, not calling you names, not having a tantrum, or regulating their feelings and emotions. What you *can* do is help guide your child to make good choices. This comes from creating connection, setting clear limits, teaching skills, and giving emotional support through unconditional love—even if you don't agree with the behavior. Connection does not equal condoning.

The Secret to Ending Power Struggles

Power struggles thrive on opposition. You have an agenda, and so does your toddler. The more you push, the more your toddler pushes back. Again, the secret to disarming these conflicts is simple yet profound: Stop trying to win. When you disengage from the struggle, you create space to do the following:

- Calm down and regulate your own emotions.
- Meet your child where they are emotionally and developmentally.
- Recognize and respect their feelings and needs.
- Move forward with a sense of empowerment rather than frustration (being in charge vs. trying to be in control).

Let's take nail clipping, for example (a power struggle I get asked about *a lot*). When it's time to clip your toddler's nails and resistance kicks in, shift the focus from "getting it done" to creating a team effort. Start by involving them in the process rather than making them a passive bystander. Hand them the clippers (or a nail file) and say, "Want to practice on me first?" Giving them a sense of control can ease anxiety and shift the dynamic from resistance to curiosity. Offer simple choices within your boundaries: "Should we start with fingers or toes? Which finger first?" This small bit of control can make a big difference.

If they're still hesitant, model the process by clipping your own nails or even your partner's while they watch. "See? It doesn't hurt." Sometimes letting them "help" or even use a nail file can build comfort and trust. To keep things light, turn the task into play: "Let's pretend the clippers are a spaceship landing on each nail!" Silly sound effects can go a long way toward defusing tension.

If all else fails, ask yourself: *Is this urgent or can it wait?* Maybe you can try again later or even clip their nails while they're asleep—without compromising their sense of bodily autonomy. And remember, skip the logic; toddlers struggle to process explanations when they're upset. Stay calm, connect with your child, and work together. You're not just clipping nails—you're building trust and fostering cooperation.

> **TODDLER TIP**
> *Take a Step Back*
>
> The next time you feel yourself being pulled into a power struggle, take a physical step back. This simple act can help you pause and disrupt your stress response and give you the mental space to choose a different response.

Seven Tools to Respond to Power Struggles

The goal in any interaction with your toddler should be to empower them, not to overpower them. Here are seven practical tools to help you navigate and disarm power struggles:

1. **Choices:** Offer your child a choice within your boundaries to give them a sense of control.
   - Example: "Would you like the red cup or the blue cup?"
2. **When/Then:** Set clear expectations without resorting to threats or bribes. This is different from a bribe, which sounds like "If you clean up the toys, I'll give you a piece of chocolate." That's dangling a reward in front of your child, then giving it for complying. When/then is about moving on to the next activity in the rhythm once the current activity is completed or the expectation is met.
   - Example: "When you wash your hands, then we can have a snack."
3. **Moving Forward:** Don't wait for your toddler to make the first move—proceed with the next task calmly.
   - Example: It's time to leave the house, so you put on your coat and shoes. Maybe you take a bag to the car. When your toddler sees you moving forward, they will likely follow due to their need for connection.
4. **Natural Consequences:** Allow your child to experience the natural outcomes of their choices, within safe limits.
   - Example: Instead of forcing your child to put on gloves in the winter, let them feel the cold and decide for themselves.
5. **Connection:** Foster cooperation through curiosity, validation, and playfulness.
   - Example: "Who do you think will make it to the bathtub first? Let's see! One, two, three, go!"
6. **Bodily Autonomy:** Encourage your child to make decisions about their body, reinforcing their ability to listen to their own needs.
   - Example: "I hear you saying you don't want to go potty before we leave. There's a potty in the car, so let me know when you need to go."
7. **Boundaries:** Look for ways to meet your child's needs within your boundaries.
   - Example: Instead of constantly telling your child to stop climbing on things, find an appropriate place for them to climb, like an outdoor play structure, bunk bed ladder, step stool, Pikler triangle, or Swedish climbing ladder.

Preventing Power Struggles

Wouldn't it be great if you could prevent power struggles before they even begin? By being proactive in these three ways, you can set the stage for smoother interactions:

1. **Use the Environment to Your Advantage:** Adjust the physical environment to meet your child's needs or to establish limits.
   - Example: If your child won't give you the toothbrush to check their teeth, give them one for each hand to hold while you use a separate one.
2. **Create Clarity Around Nonnegotiables:** Define what's truly nonnegotiable so you can be flexible when appropriate.
   - Example: Brushing teeth is nonnegotiable, but wearing pajamas might not be.
3. **Release the Pressure:** Children often take action when they don't feel forced or backed into a corner.
   - Example: Instead of saying, "You have to go potty before we go outside," try, "There's the potty. It's here when you need it."

TODDLER TIP
Say Yes

If you find yourself saying no all the time, it can create more power struggles because toddlers crave a sense of control. Look for moments when you can say yes, even if it feels a bit inconvenient, as long as it's within your boundaries.

Overusing *no* and *stop* to set limits can trigger your toddler's natural drive to assert their independence, making them more defiant. Save these words for dangerous situations when you need

> your child to listen immediately. This keeps *no* meaningful and helps maintain a more cooperative dynamic.

A New Approach to Power Struggles

It takes two people to be in a power struggle, but it only takes one to step back and change the dynamic. As the adult, you have the power to disengage and model a different way of handling conflict. Remember, progress doesn't mean perfection. You're not striving for flawlessness—you're learning and growing alongside your child. There is usually more than one way to get to the same outcome, so be flexible and get creative to meet your child's needs within your boundaries.

When the sun peeks through your blinds tomorrow morning, you have a choice. You can brace yourself for another day of tug-of-war, or you can embrace the opportunity to connect, teach, and grow alongside your child. When you disarm the power struggle, you're not just avoiding conflict—you're building a foundation of trust and cooperation that will serve you both for years to come.

FAQs

How do I pick and choose my battles with my child?

Power struggles often arise because both parents and toddlers have legitimate needs. Parents want to maintain control and create structure, while toddlers are wired to assert their independence and explore their ability to influence the world around them. Understanding this dynamic helps you approach challenging moments with empathy and creativity rather than seeing them as battles to win.

This is why I don't recommend thinking of parenting in terms of "picking and choosing battles." This mindset frames interactions as a win-or-lose power struggle, leaving you either giving in to your child or digging your heels in to "win" at all costs. Instead, shift the focus from battling to meeting needs and problem-solving.

Ask yourself the following questions:

- What's the goal here?
- Are there multiple ways to achieve this goal?
- Does it have to happen right now, or can it wait?
- Am I prepared to follow through while still considering my child's needs?

My toddler hates the car seat, and it always seems like a battle to get her in. What should I do?

Toddlers don't like being restricted—they're wired to experiment, explore, and, most of all, move! To avoid a stressful struggle, try heading to the car five to ten minutes early so you're not under time pressure. Give your child a sense of control and help them feel powerful: "Show me how this buckle works—I need your help!" Keep the process engaging by having fun toys in the car and using a simple when/then statement: "When you get in, then we can turn on your favorite song!"

Offer choices to foster cooperation: "Do you want to climb into the car seat yourself, or do you want me to help you?" But if your child resists and you're out of time, you may have to override their protests to keep them safe. In these moments, be calm, clear, and validating: "It's time to get in the car seat. I hear that you don't want to, and it's time for us to leave. I'm going to help you get buckled." Acknowledge their feelings and do your best to keep the interaction positive, reinforcing that you're on their team—even when you have to take charge.

Chapter 28

HANDLING TRANSITIONS

It's time to leave the playground, and your toddler is completely immersed in their world—sliding, climbing, and fully absorbed in the magic of play. Then comes the dreaded moment: "It's time to go." From your toddler's perspective, this can feel like a jarring interruption. Think about it: Toddlers have very little control over their days. They're constantly being told where to go, what to do, and when to do it. They don't grasp the abstract nature of time like adults do—they live fully in the present, not worrying about the errands or schedule ahead.

So when we ask them to stop their fun and shift gears—whether that's interrupting their play or simply asking them to participate in routine activities like eating breakfast or getting dressed—it's no surprise they resist. Transitions feel uncertain, and for toddlers, uncertainty can feel like chaos, often leading to power struggles and tantrums when their play or routines are disrupted. But with a little preparation, connection, and creativity, you can guide your child through transitions with less resistance and more cooperation.

7 Tips for Navigating Transitions

Transition Tip 1: Avoid Yes/No Questions

When adults speak to other adults, it's common to hear directives formed as questions. At work, you might hear someone say, "Do you mind printing this out?" It's often meant to soften a request that isn't actually a request. We understand the context as adults. Toddlers, on the other hand, don't understand contextual language. They hear us giving an option when we don't mean to. You say, "Are you ready to brush your teeth?" and you're met with "*No!*" because your toddler hears you *literally*. When we ask yes/no questions, we unintentionally set ourselves up for a power struggle.

Transition Tip 2: Offer Choices Within Boundaries

Choices give toddlers a sense of control, which is exactly what they're craving during transitions. But here's the trick: The choices should be within your personal boundaries. For example, when it's time to leave the house, you could say, "Do you want to wear your sandals or sneakers?" When bath time rolls around, offer, "Do you want to race me to the bathroom or have a piggyback ride?"

By offering these choices, you're giving your child control without relinquishing your boundaries. It's a win-win: They feel empowered, and you're still in charge of the bigger picture. However, even when you give two options in an effort to partner with a child, you may still hear no. Often when your child says no to your choices, they have a plan. Get curious about their idea. You don't have to agree with or go with your child's plan, but just simply letting them express themselves creates a connection.

Transition Tip 3: Use a Visual Timer

Time is an abstract concept for toddlers—they don't know how long five minutes is or why they need to stop playing right now. A visual timer can make the idea of time more concrete for them. It gives them a sense of how much time they have left, reducing the anxiety that comes with the unknown.

You can set a visual timer when transitioning from one activity to another, like from playtime to lunch or from watching a show to getting ready for dinner. When your toddler can see time passing visually, it helps them understand that this change isn't sudden, and they have time to adjust.

Transition Tip 4: Give Advanced Notice—But Make It Connect

Going over the plan for the day can help your toddler feel secure and reduce the stress of transitions. Toddlers thrive when they know what's coming next, so taking a moment to map out the day for them is powerful: "After breakfast, we'll play for a bit, then head to the store. After your nap, we'll go to the park." Simple, clear, and predictable—it helps them see the day as a sequence of manageable events.

When it comes to transitions, a five-minute warning can make all the difference—if it's done with connection. Shouting "Five more minutes!" from across the room rarely lands the way we hope. Instead, meet your child where they are. Get down on their level, make eye contact, and use a warm, inviting tone to say, "In five minutes, we'll clean up and get ready for lunch." Engage their attention fully—this moment of connection is key.

Make the warning tangible. Use a hand signal, hold up five fingers, or even better, set a visual timer they can see. This gives them something concrete to latch onto, bridging the gap between abstract time and their current focus.

Transition Tip 5: Bridge the Gap

For your toddler, stopping play to move on to something else can feel deeply frustrating because their agenda is play—not whatever you're asking them to do. This is where a "transitional object" can be a game changer—a special toy, lovey, or some of the items they were playing with. For example, the other day my son was playing with new stickers when it was time to go. My husband said, "Time to leave. Go get your shoes," and my son said no. This is a classic example of meeting your child with logic instead of where they are. I went up to my son with a small bag and said, "Those stickers are so fun! Let's put them in this bag with your paper and take them to the coffee shop." His face lit up, he put them in, and we left without a fuss because I met him where he was.

Transition Tip 6: Make It a Playful Game

Sometimes the best way to get through a transition is to make it fun. Turn the mundane into something playful. Instead of saying, "It's time to go," try, "Let's see if we can hop like bunnies all the way to the car!" or "Stand on my feet and we will walk together." Or if it's time to clean up, challenge them to a race: "I wonder if you can put all the blocks away before the timer runs out. Let's try it!"

Transition Tip 7: Allow Space for Emotions

Even with all the best strategies, your toddler might still struggle with transitions. And that's okay. Sometimes what they need most is space to express their frustration. Give them room to feel upset, and validate their emotions without trying to "fix" them. Remember, emotions aren't good or bad. They are reactions to the situation.

Instead of trying to force happiness or compliance, acknowledge their feelings: "It's upsetting when it's time to leave the playground. It's hard to stop when you're having so much fun." By validating their emotions, you're showing them that it's okay to feel what they feel. This helps them build emotional resilience and makes transitions smoother in the long run.

At the end of the day, transitions are a part of life, and while they might be tough for toddlers, they're also opportunities for growth. By offering connection, choices, and understanding, you're helping your child learn how to navigate change with confidence—and without the power struggles. With the right tools and a little creativity, you can transform even the most dreaded transitions into moments of cooperation and connection.

FAQs

My toddler struggles leaving the park and the children's museum. I know they are having fun, but when it's time to go, it's time to go! How do I help them make this transition better?

Leaving a fun place like the park or museum can be tough for toddlers, but you can ease the transition by connecting with their feelings: "You love it here, and it's hard to leave." Set a clear limit: "It's time to go," and offer playful choices to give them a sense of control: "Do you want a piggyback ride or to race to the car?" If they don't choose, calmly follow through, remembering that tears are a normal part of processing big emotions. "Looks like you are having trouble choosing. I'm going to carry you to the car now."

I'm struggling to get my toddler dressed in the mornings. It always turns into a power struggle. What can I do?

Morning dressing battles with toddlers often stem from their desire for independence (and at times their fear of separation, if they have to go to school or daycare). If you've offered two choices, like "Do you want the blue shirt or the red one?" and they still resist, try saying, "What's your idea?" instead of, "Just pick one or I'll choose for you."

If they refuse both options—"No, I don't want them!"—stay calm and set a gentle boundary: "Sounds like you don't want to choose today. You can try again tomorrow. I'm going to choose the red one, and now we're going to get dressed. Do you want to put on the shirt or pants first?"

There might be some strong feelings as a result. Meltdowns happen when toddlers don't get their way or feel like they are not able to choose what they want, and meltdowns are okay. They are learning how to express their feelings about a situation that is out of their control. It's important to recognize the validity of their feelings and move forward from there.

Chapter 29

BUILDING YOUR CHILD'S CONFIDENCE

Every parent dreams of raising a child who grows up to be a confident, resilient adult—someone who faces the world with grit, grace, and an unshakable belief in themself. But that kind of confidence doesn't just appear out of nowhere. It's forged in the fires of first challenges—first steps, first words, first attempts at independence—and each of these milestones is an opportunity for your child to learn something vital: *that they are capable.*

Confidence isn't about fearlessness. It's about trusting they can try, fail, and try again. It's the foundation of resilience—the ability to adapt, manage big emotions, and keep going when things don't go as planned.

Building resilience means walking the tightrope of parenting's greatest dilemma—when to protect and when to let go. It's about knowing when to step in with support and when to step back to make space. True confidence isn't built through praise or overprotection; it's created through effort, risk-taking, and learning from mistakes. And your toddler learns that best with you cheering them on every step of the way.

> **TODDLER TIP**
> *Avoid Negative Talk*
>
> Refrain from talking about kids in a negative way in front of them, whether it's to your parenting partner or even the pediatrician. Toddlers internalize what they hear us say about them. From time to time, you might consider letting them purposely overhear you saying something positive about them to your parenting partner or even their lovey.

Unlearning Labels and Rethinking Praise

"You're so cute!"

"I love your little toes."

"Good job!"

How many times a day do these words spill out of your mouth, directed at the little bundle of energy? These are the phrases we use to express our love, admiration, and pride. And why not? It feels good to tell our children how wonderful they are, and it feels even better to see their faces light up in response! Praise is powerful—it's a bridge to connection, a way to affirm our love, and a tool to help our children build a positive self-image.

But as with any powerful tool, how we use praise can shape the foundations we lay for our children's self-worth and confidence. There's a subtle but crucial difference between praise that grows confidence and praise that inadvertently narrows a child's understanding of their value. It's tempting to celebrate every adorable thing they do, but when praise focuses only on qualities like being "cute" or "smart," or only on outcomes ("Good job!"), it can send the message that their value lies in what they achieve or how others see them.

Research shows that praising or labeling children with fixed traits, even positive ones like "smart," can limit their potential.[1] Kids internalize these labels, which can create pressure to live up to them. A child who hears "You're so smart!" might shy away from challenges for fear of failing and losing that label. Instead of seeing mistakes as part of growth, they may stick to safe, easy tasks where they're sure to succeed.

This is especially important during the toddler years, when children are developing their sense of self for the first time. Labels—both positive and negative—become part of their identity. For example, a toddler praised only for doing a good job may start to believe that mistakes make them less lovable or capable, reinforcing perfectionistic tendencies.

This doesn't mean we should stop praising our children altogether or that saying "Good job!" sometimes is wrong—far from it! The key is to shift the focus of our praise overall to emphasize effort, process, and specific feedback. This type of praise encourages a growth mindset, a concept popularized by psychologist Carol Dweck. In her research, Dweck found that children who are praised for their efforts and strategies are more likely to develop a growth mindset, where they see their abilities as something they can develop through hard work and perseverance. In contrast, children who are praised for innate qualities, like intelligence or talent, may develop a fixed mindset, where they believe their abilities are static and unchangeable.[2]

So how do we break the cycle of labels and help our children build confidence and resilience? The key is to focus on the process, effort, and growth, rather than the outcome or static traits. Here is what that looks like in practice:

- **Praise the Process:** Instead of saying, "You're so smart!" when your child solves a puzzle, try saying, "I noticed how hard you worked to figure that out. You didn't give up, even when it was tricky! You did it!" This emphasizes the effort and perseverance they displayed, rather than labeling them as inherently smart. When you praise the process instead of the outcome, you help your toddler
    - build intrinsic motivation and confidence in their abilities,
    - develop problem-solving skills and creativity,

- foster a growth mindset, where challenges are opportunities to learn,
- reduce the need for external approval or validation, and
- emphasize effort over outcome or perfection, teaching them that mistakes are part of the journey.

- **Acknowledge the Effort:** When your child tries something new, whether it's learning to tie their shoes or drawing a picture, focus on the effort they put into it. "I saw all the concentration you put into tying your shoes all by yourself! You're getting better every day."
- **Celebrate Growth:** When your child makes progress in a skill, celebrate the improvement. You might say, "Wow, you've learned so many new words this week! Your reading is getting stronger because you keep practicing," or "Wow, you raised your hand to hit me, then you decided not to. Look at all the self-control you are developing," or "Wow, look how high you are swinging! Your legs are getting so strong!"
- **Give Specific Feedback:** Instead of always relying on nonspecific feedback, focus on acknowledging specific behaviors by describing what you see. "Thanks for putting your plate in the sink." "You put all of your toys in the bin!"

SCRIPTS FOR COMMUNICATION
Praising

Focus on praising the effort, process, or action instead of the outcome to build up your child's self-esteem.

Avoid Saying: "You're so cute!"
Try Saying: "You make the world a better place by being you" or "I love you just the way you are."

> **Avoid Saying:** "You're so smart."
> **Try Saying:** "That was challenging and you kept trying!"
>
> **Avoid Saying:** "Good job!"
> **Try Saying:** "Thank you for (insert action)" or "You (insert positive behavior)!"

Building Confidence Through Independence

Supporting your toddler's budding independence isn't just about letting them do things on their own; it's about giving them the tools to feel confident and capable. Research backs this up—when kids feel capable, their confidence soars, and with it comes the pride of knowing *I did that!*[3]

And here's the best part: Every challenge they face with your gentle support helps build resilience. Imagine your child is learning to get dressed independently. At first, you might lay out their clothes, talk them through the process, and assist with tricky parts like buttoning or tying shoes. Over time, as they become more familiar with the steps, you gradually reduce your involvement, allowing them to take on more responsibility until they can do it entirely on their own.

So how can you support your toddler's independence in meaningful, practical ways?

Make Their World Accessible

Creating a toddler-friendly environment helps children feel empowered to explore and take charge of their daily tasks. Here are a couple of easy ways to give them opportunities:

- Use a **toddler tower** to give them safe access to counters for helping in the kitchen and sinks for personal care in the bathroom.
- Hang coats, books, and mirrors at their height so they can reach and use them independently.

Make Things Understandable

Toddlers thrive on clarity and structure. Make routines and tasks easy to follow with these tips:

- Use a **visual routine chart** to outline morning or bedtime steps, helping them know what comes next without constant reminders.
- Use **visual cues** like stickers to help them distinguish between right and left shoes or labels with pictures to show where toys and clothing belong.

Allow Room for Mistakes

Failure is a natural part of learning, and allowing your toddler to make mistakes teaches them valuable problem-solving skills. Whether it's spilling water while pouring or struggling to zip a jacket, step back and let them try. When they succeed, the sense of achievement is that much sweeter. Here's how you can create opportunities for them:

- **Break Tasks into Manageable Steps:** If your child is learning a complex skill, break it down into smaller, more manageable steps. Celebrate each success along the way to keep them motivated.
- **Gradually Reduce Support:** As your child becomes more confident and capable, gradually reduce the level of support you provide. This might mean stepping back physically, offering fewer verbal prompts, or encouraging them to take on more responsibility.
- **Model Positive Self-Talk:** Modeling positive self-talk teaches your toddler how to approach challenges with self-compassion and resilience. When you reframe your own mistakes with phrases like "I'll try again!" or "This is tricky, but I can figure it out," you're showing them that setbacks are opportunities to learn and grow.

Those little wins after a stumble—zipping their jacket, stacking the block tower again after it falls—teach them that persistence pays off. By fostering independence, you're not only helping your toddler master the tasks of today but also equipping them with the confidence, resilience, and determination they'll need to thrive tomorrow.

> **TODDLER TIP**
> *Nurture Independence*
>
> Support your toddler in feeling capable by allowing them to do what you would normally do for them because you can do it faster and better. Toddlers learn best through experience and need opportunities to practice. Practice makes progress, not perfection!

Raising Confident, Resilient Children

As you navigate the journey of parenthood, remember that the words you choose, the opportunities you provide, and the support you offer all play a crucial role in shaping your child's confidence and resilience. By offering praise that emphasizes effort and growth, encouraging risky play, and supporting independence, you're helping them build a strong foundation for a lifetime of self-confidence and success.

And as you do this, keep in mind that your own journey as a parent is one of growth and learning too. Embrace the challenges, celebrate the successes, and know that every small step you take is helping your child become the confident, resilient individual they're meant to be.

FAQs

Why does my toddler lack confidence in social situations?

What might look like a lack of confidence could actually be that your child is more reserved and slower to warm up. Being slow to warm up is part of their temperament and doesn't mean they lack confidence. (See chapter 41, "Supporting a Slow-to-Warm-Up (Shy) Child," for more.)

Is it bad to say "Good job"?

Absolutely not! As a parent, I invite you to stop thinking about parenting strategies as good or bad. Instead, start thinking about whether or not they are developmentally appropriate, effective, and supportive of your family values. You aren't going to "ruin" your child by saying "Good job!" However, it's not the most effective way to build your child's confidence.

My toddler is in a "Why?" stage and is constantly asking questions. How do I handle this?

When your toddler is asking a question that they are confident they can work out, try simply replying with, "I'm curious. What do you think?" Some toddlers ask parents questions to capture their attention. If your instincts are telling you this is the reason beneath the behavior, I suggest connecting with your toddler in an intentional way. Make eye contact and get on their level as you ask them this question and remain engaged while they speak.

If my toddler is struggling to do something, should I step in and do it for them?

If your child isn't overly frustrated, then give them the space to keep trying and work through it. If you need to support them, you might say, "I wonder what would happen if you . . ." If your child gets very frustrated, then validate them. "That's so frustrating! You are trying to tie your shoes and it's not working the way you thought." Then either suggest a break or say, "I wonder what we can do to make this better." You can also model the skill for your child and help them practice.

Part 4

THE PHYSICAL TODDLER

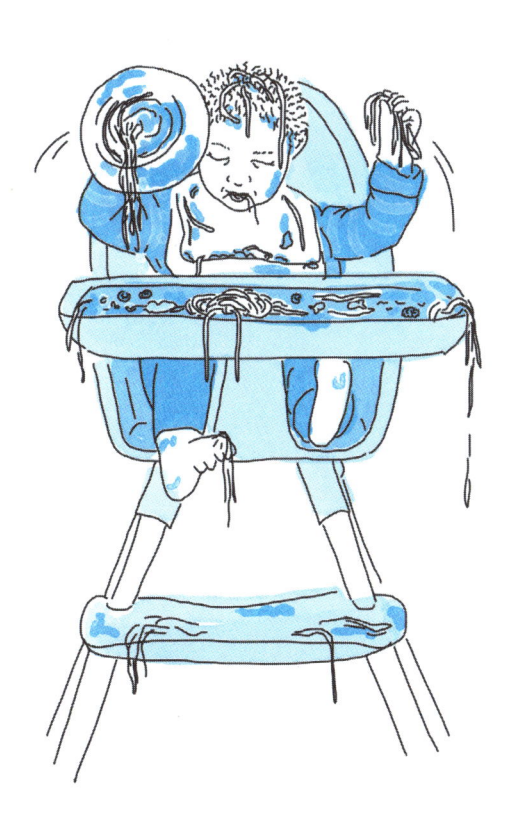

Chapter 30

CULTIVATING CONSENT AND BODY-SAFETY SKILLS

Consent isn't just for grown-ups—it's a vital part of all healthy relationships, whether you're navigating the complexities of adulthood or guiding a toddler through their first few years of life.

Yep, you heard that right. Teaching your child about consent starts in the toddler years, and it's one of the most empowering gifts you can offer your child.

Picture this: It's the holidays and your aunt Sue walks through the front door holding her famous green bean casserole. Your toddler stands next to you, eyes wide, looking at relatives they barely know. Then Aunt Sue, with all her love and warmth, opens her arms wide for a hug.

You feel it—the internal tug-of-war. You don't want to hurt anyone's feelings, but then, there's your child, clutching your leg, unsure and not quite ready to leap into the arms of someone who is essentially a stranger. And this is where a pivotal lesson begins: teaching consent, right here, in this small yet powerful moment.

I get it. You're thinking, *But my family will insist on a hug and be so hurt when my child refuses!* It's tempting to brush off your toddler's hesitation. After all, Aunt Sue is family, and what harm could a little hug do? But for your child, that moment of hesitation is their way of asserting, in the only way they know how, that their body is their own. They're telling you, even without words, that they need control over when and how they show affection.

Instead of nudging your child forward with a quiet, "Go on. It's just a hug," you kneel and ask, "How would you like to say hi to Aunt Sue? Would you like to give a hug, a wave, or maybe a high five?" Suddenly, the power is in your toddler's hands, and they get to choose how they interact. Aunt Sue might be a little disappointed, maybe even confused, but you stand firm, gently reminding her, "We're teaching consent, and it's important for them to choose."

By doing this, you're teaching your child that *their voice matters* and that they are in charge of their own body—even when you are the one introducing them to new people. You're sending the powerful message that they don't have to please others at the expense of their own needs or feelings of discomfort. Remember: Your child gets to decide when and how they show affection.

Keeping Bodies Safe

Consent education isn't just about teaching toddlers how to interact respectfully with others—it's a critical tool for protecting them from harm. In the United States, one in four girls and one in six boys experience sexual abuse, and those are just the reported cases.[1] The real numbers are likely higher, with many instances going unreported. In some parts of the world, these statistics are even more alarming. What's more, 90 percent of abusers are someone the child knows, whether it's a family member, family friend, or peer—often in familiar settings like daycare or a family member's home.[2]

As your child's guide and primary protector, it's your job to recognize the signs of grooming, identify safe and unsafe individuals, and take proactive steps to keep your child safe. Abusers often rely on manipulation, not physical force, using grooming techniques to gain a child's trust and ensure their silence.

Common Grooming Behaviors
- **One-on-One Time Requests:** Offering free babysitting or insisting on spending extra alone time with your child.

- **Lavish Gifts and Excessive Attention:** Providing extravagant presents or constant attention to build dependence and loyalty.
- **Secret Keeping:** Encouraging your child to keep secrets from you.
- **Excessive Physical Play:** Engaging in frequent hands-on activities like roughhousing, tickling, or extended cuddling.

As your child's guide and protector, it's your responsibility to recognize red flags, identify unsafe individuals, and take proactive steps to keep your child safe. It's never too early to start these conversations. By teaching your child about consent, boundaries, and safety rules, you're equipping them with tools that go far beyond today's playground dynamics; they're gaining lifelong skills to protect themself.

Key Safety Rules
- **Keep Doors Open:** When playing with other kids or during playdates, ensure doors stay open so activities are visible.
- **Know Their Whereabouts:** Stay aware of where your child is, especially during holiday gatherings or events where supervision might be inconsistent.
- **Teach Boundaries:** Show your child how to say no confidently. Use role-playing exercises to practice refusing unwanted physical contact, like hugs or tickling.
- **Explain Consent:** Use simple terms to explain consent: "You get to choose if someone can touch you." Then practice by modeling consent: "Can I give you a kiss goodnight?" Respect your child's answer.
- **Teach Safe vs. Unsafe Touch:** Explain where it's okay to be touched and where it is not. Use clear, age-appropriate language to make this concept understandable. "No one touches your penis but you, *and* you don't touch anyone else's penis. No one else should see or touch this part of your body because it's private."

Most of all, normalize conversations about consent and safety at home. This ensures your child feels safe coming to you with *anything*, no matter how small or serious. Open, ongoing discussions lay the foundation for trust, empowering your child to share concerns, seek help, and feel confident asserting their boundaries whenever needed.

> ### TODDLER TIP
> *Avoid Secrets*
>
> Refrain from asking your toddler to keep secrets from another parent or adult. Even seemingly harmless phrases like "Don't tell Mommy I let you eat chips" are not recommended because they normalize secret keeping. Teaching kids to keep secrets—no matter how harmless they seem—can set a dangerous precedent. Predators often rely on children's willingness to keep secrets to hide harmful behavior.
>
> As your toddler gets older, you can help them learn the difference between a secret and a surprise. A secret is something you're asked to never tell anyone, and it can make you feel uncomfortable, worried, or sad. A surprise is something exciting that brings joy and happiness, and you'll tell someone about it after hiding it for a short time.

Using Anatomically Correct Names

I remember hearing the story of a three-year-old girl who would tell her teachers that her uncle "eats her cookie." The teachers didn't think anything of it and even encouraged her to keep baking cookies. It wasn't until the girl's mom came in, worried about a rash on her "cookie," that they realized what the child was actually trying to communicate.

This heartbreaking example highlights why it's so important to use anatomically correct names for body parts with your toddler. When children learn that their vulva and vagina, or penis and scrotum, are just as normal as their legs, eyes, hands, and feet, they're less likely to view these parts as secret or "bad," empowering them to talk openly and accurately, without shame or embarrassment. While genitals are private in terms of touching or exposing, they're not so private that we can't talk about them. Bath time, diaper changes, and getting dressed are a great time to practice. By normalizing these conversations, you're equipping your child with the confidence and tools they need to navigate their world safely and confidently. Teaching proper names lays the groundwork for understanding boundaries and consent, which can prevent abuse. If something inappropriate happens, they are better equipped to communicate clearly and be understood.

Depending on how you grew up, using these words might feel awkward or uncomfortable at first. That's okay. Acknowledge those feelings and give yourself time to process them. Start by reading your child books that teach consent. The more you use these words, the easier it becomes—and the more your child learns that their body is nothing to be embarrassed about.

> For my list of favorite toddler books on this topic of consent, visit transformingtoddlerhood.com/bookresources.

Normalizing Consent and Bodily Autonomy in Everyday Life

Young children are the most vulnerable to abuse—especially kids who are preverbal. Toddlers can be easy targets because they are dependent on adults to get their physical and emotional needs met, so they are quick to trust. Consent is a vital part of all healthy relationships in adulthood *and* toddlerhood. You can never talk about consent too early or too often.

So what does consent look like when your little one is still mastering the art of stringing together sentences? It's about giving permission for something to happen, especially when it comes to touch. When it comes to setting boundaries with others and respecting the boundaries of others, try to keep it as simple as possible. "No one can touch your body without your permission. If someone touches you and you don't want them to, say no. If you're touching someone and they say no, stop immediately. No means no."

The key is allowing your toddler to say no without making it "bad." It's about supporting them in setting boundaries. Whether it's during toilet learning, greeting friends and relatives, tickling games, mealtimes, or any other physical interaction, the following everyday moments are ripe with opportunities to practice consent:

- **Toilet Learning:** Instead of saying, "Be a good girl/boy and go to the bathroom before we go," try saying, "It's time to leave. Let's take a moment to try to go potty before leaving. It's okay if you don't go pee." Respect their response, even if it's a no. This teaches them that their body cues are important and that they have a say in what happens to their body.
- **Greeting Friends and Relatives:** Help your toddler hold boundaries with adults, siblings, and peers. "She doesn't want to hug you right now." Instead of insisting on a hug or a kiss, offer alternatives. "Grandma is here. Would you like to give Grandma a hug, a high five, or just wave hello?" This gives them the power to decide how they want to interact physically.
- **Tickling:** This is a touchy subject because it can dysregulate kids and make it hard for them to say stop. It's best practice not to tickle kids. If you want to play this way, always ask, "Can I tickle you?" before diving in. If they say stop, stop immediately. This simple act reinforces that they have control over their body and that their words are respected.
- **Mealtimes:** When it comes to feeding, respect their cues. If they turn their head away or push the spoon away, don't force them to eat. This teaches them to listen to their body's signals. Instead of saying, "Be a good girl/boy and eat your lunch," try saying, "You can eat the rest of your lunch if you feel hungry. If you're not hungry, you can be done."

- **Physical Interactions:** Whether it's brushing their hair or wiping their face, ask first. "Can I wipe your face?" It may seem small, but it's teaching them that their consent is needed.

Teach your child that *no means no*. Show them that their boundaries matter by respecting their wishes when they say they don't want to be tickled, hugged, kissed, or tossed in the air. Practice with them—encourage them to say "no" or "stop" confidently and demonstrate how to respond by immediately stopping what you're doing.

Equally important, teach them to respect others' boundaries. You can also model this when you set your own boundaries with your child. Explain that when someone else says "no" or "stop," they must stop tickling, touching, or roughhousing right away. These simple lessons help your child understand that everyone has the right to set boundaries and have them respected.

Teaching bodily autonomy supports kids in learning to listen to their bodies and trust themselves. The culture of creating compliance goes against this by teaching kids to people-please over listening to their own feelings, emotions, needs, and bodies. It's about empowering them to set boundaries, listen to their inner voice, and communicate confidently. And most importantly, it's about showing them that their body, their voice, and their feelings matter. By practicing consent now, you're giving them the tools they need to navigate the world with confidence, respect, and self-assurance.

So start the conversations. Normalize the words. Practice the scripts. And watch as your little one grows into a person who knows their worth, trusts their instincts, and respects the boundaries of others—because they learned it all from you.

FAQs

How can I talk to my toddler about tricky people without scaring them?

It's about empowering them with tools, not filling them with fear. Say something like this: "If someone asks you to go somewhere with them and it doesn't feel right, or if they ask you to keep a secret, you can always tell me. Your body belongs to you, and you get to decide who gives you hugs or holds your hand. If anyone makes you feel uncomfortable, even if you know them, you should tell a grown-up you trust."

Make it clear that tricky people aren't always strangers; they can be someone they know. What matters is trusting their gut feeling—kids are amazing at reading people when we encourage them to listen to themselves.

I found my toddler and her friend with their clothes off showing their body parts to each other. No one was touching each other, but clearly, they should have their clothes on. How should I handle this?

It's normal for toddlers to be curious about their bodies and the bodies of others. Stay neutral and clear. You might say, "It's time to put our clothes back on. Clothes stay on during playdates." Then leave it at that and keep a close eye on them moving forward. Later, you can have a discussion about privacy and consent with your toddler. Continue these conversations often and allow your child to ask questions. Keep the conversation free of blame, shame, guilt, judgment, and fear.

I want to practice bodily autonomy with my toddler but struggle when they won't get into their car seat or take their medicine. How should I handle this?

Giving kids bodily autonomy not only helps them trust their bodies but also can keep them safe from predators. As much as we want to practice bodily autonomy with our toddler all the time, there are some moments when we have to override our toddler's bodily autonomy because it's our job to keep them safe and healthy.

My toddler keeps touching their genitals. What should I do?

It's completely normal for toddlers to explore their genitals—it's no different to them than discovering their fingers, toes, or ears. This behavior isn't sexual; it's often driven by curiosity or comfort and may even help regulate their nervous system. If your toddler starts touching themselves, avoid making a big deal about it and set boundaries as needed. Shaming or scolding can make them feel bad about their body and less likely to come to you if something happens to them. Instead, use these moments to teach about privacy. If it happens in public, calmly redirect their attention to another activity. Reinforce the important message that no one else, not even adults, is allowed to touch their private parts. By approaching the topic with calmness and care, you create an open, shame-free environment where your child feels safe discussing their body with you.

Chapter 31

STOPPING AGGRESSIVE BEHAVIOR

It was an ordinary morning, and I was making my usual cup of matcha, savoring the promise of caffeine while my little one stood on his kitchen toddler tower. As I poured the milk into the frother, his eyes lit up. "Push button!" he demanded, bouncing with excitement.

"Yes, in just a minute," I said as I got everything in place, but before I could process what happened next—*whack!*—a tiny hand landed smack dab on my forehead.

When this happens a parent's first instinct may be to scold or react sharply. But the key in these shocking (sometimes very painful) moments is to pause, take a deep breath, and consider the situation. The reality? This wasn't personal. It wasn't even "bad" behavior. He was eager and frustrated, and didn't have the words and patience to express it.

But then something unexpected happened—his face crumpled. He realized he had hit me and burst into tears, overwhelmed by what he had done. His little hands reached up, seeking comfort, as if saying, "I didn't mean to—I don't know what to do with all these feelings."

In that moment, I saw his struggle clearly. He wasn't just mad because he couldn't push the button—he was also scared and confused by his own actions. Sometimes this shows up as tears and other times as laughter. It doesn't mean your child thinks hitting is funny. It means they are dysregulated. Toddlers are still figuring out how to navigate a big, overwhelming world with very few tools at their disposal, and their biggest fear is losing our unconditional love and acceptance. Sometimes they lash out—not to be cruel, but because they can't yet express their needs, emotions, or sensory overload with words. In fact, your toddler's developmental drive and their feelings, emotions, desires, and unmet needs are often stronger than their impulse control and ability to regulate themself.

> ## TODDLER TIP
> *Reframe Aggressive Behavior*
>
> Of all the concerns I hear from worried parents and caregivers, concerns about aggressive behaviors are the ones that come up most often (and with most alarm). When your toddler hits, bites, kicks, or throws, they are doing just that. *Aggressive* is a label we place on the behavior as an interpretation, and that judgment doesn't do us any favors. Oftentimes it can fuel our stress response and cause us to spiral.
>
> The truth is these behaviors don't mean your child is bad or that they are going to grow up to be a bully. Aggressive behaviors are in fact—you guessed it!—developmentally appropriate behaviors. I invite you to flip the narrative and either describe the behavior like a sportscaster—"He hit me on the forehead"—or call them out-of-control behaviors, which more accurately describes what is happening.

Reasons for Out-of-Control Behavior

Toddlers are *built to move*. Their little bodies are designed for action—running, climbing, jumping, and, yes, sometimes hitting, kicking, biting, or throwing. When big emotions like frustration, fear, sadness, or even excitement bubble up inside them, those emotions have to go somewhere. Since toddlers haven't yet mastered the skills to express themselves with words or regulate their feelings, their emotions often spill out physically. *Most* (if not *all*) children experiment with using these behaviors at some point in toddlerhood.

Here are the different developmental phases toddlers go through when it comes to out-of-control behavior.

Younger Toddlers: Experimentation

At this age, hitting, biting, and throwing are often experimental. They're learning cause and effect: *What happens if I hit? What happens if I bite?* They're also figuring out how to interact with the world. Redirecting them toward acceptable outlets by saying things like "You can hit this pillow when you're mad" or "You can bite this teething ring" teaches them appropriate ways to channel their energy. Also, modeling gentle touch can be helpful.

Older Toddlers: Coping Mechanisms

As toddlers get older, these behaviors can become an ingrained response to stress, frustration, or feeling out of control. By this stage, they may be using hitting or biting as a way to communicate needs or manage overwhelming emotions. Imagine shaking up a bottle of soda and popping the cap—*boom!* That release of built-up pressure is exactly what happens when toddlers lash out. This is when teaching alternative coping strategies, setting limits, and modeling problem-solving become critical. They're not trying to be "bad"—they're trying to find effective ways to communicate. Also, children with speech delay and sensory processing challenges tend to have more out-of-control behaviors and tantrums.

Think about some of the ways adults handle stress:

- We exercise.
- We vent to a friend.
- We take deep breaths or step outside for air.
- We sit on the porch with a cup of tea (or something stronger).

Toddlers don't have the same coping tools we have. What they *do* have is their bodies. Hitting, biting, kicking, or throwing things becomes an instinctive release when emotions overflow. These behaviors aren't premeditated—they're impulsive reactions driven by an undeveloped ability to self-regulate.

Knowing this helps us shift our perspective from seeing it as a personal attack to recognizing it as a sign that something inside them needs help working its way out.

> **TODDLER TIP**
> *Create a Bridge*
>
> Meet your toddler's need for physical release while staying within your boundaries. If they feel like hitting, offer something safe to hit—a pillow, cushion, or soft toy. This creates a bridge from hitting people to using appropriate outlets, eventually leading to practicing calming techniques. It's all about giving them a safe way to work through big emotions while building better coping skills.

What the Out-of-Control Behavior Is Communicating

Now that we know all behavior is communication, it's important to get curious about and address the feeling, emotion, need, or desire at the root of the behavior instead of punishing your child for having a developmentally appropriate behavior. Addressing the root of the behavior is what transforms behavior. Here are some of the common root causes for aggressive behavior:

- **Defending Self or Others:** A toddler may hit or bite another child who has taken their toy away to say, "That's not okay."

- **Expressing the Need for Personal Space:** They may use out-of-control behavior as a way to set a boundary with another child who is in their personal space.
- **Bidding for Connection:** They need you or are seeking connection but are having a difficult time saying it.
- **Expressing Big Feelings or Physical Needs:** They may be experiencing anger or frustration or be hungry or tired.
- **Reacting to a Limit:** It can be hard for them to accept the limits we set. They are confronted with the fact they aren't in control, and they will go through a process of communicating their feelings and emotions before they accept the limit.
- **Feeling Overstimulated:** Whether it's sounds, bright lights, or feeling excited, toddlers can be sensorily overstimulated as well as emotionally overstimulated, even by what we might label as positive emotions such as excitement or happiness.
- **Experimenting:** They could be experimenting to see how we react and what our response is. They can also be experimenting with their body. Toddlers are learning about what their bodies are capable of and learning new physical skills all the time.
- **Adjusting to Changes:** When a toddler experiences big life changes such as a new sibling, starting school, parents getting divorced, or moving, it can be very unsettling for them, and these behaviors can increase as they adjust.
- **Imitating Other Children:** Toddlers are little sponges who are learning how to be and act in this world, which makes them very impressionable to what they see others do, including characters in shows.
- **Seeking Oral-Motor Stimulation:** Some kids are sensory seekers and need sensory input to feel regulated and be at their emotional equilibrium. Biting is one way they accomplish this.

While it may be challenging to pinpoint the root of the behavior, it's our job as parents to get curious. We may not always know the *exact* underlying thing our child is trying to communicate (or the perfect response to it)—and that's okay! Curiosity is *always* the best place to start when addressing challenging behavior.

Responding to Out-of-Control Behavior

Now, you might be wondering, *What response is appropriate and will convey that the behavior is unacceptable?*

First of all, know that punishment doesn't solve hitting, biting, or kicking. Lecturing a toddler, yelling, or putting them in time-out—or using shame, blame, guilt, judgment, or fear—won't teach a toddler how *not* to hit, bite, kick, or throw. Sure, these things might end the behavior *in the moment*, but they don't change the behavior long term. Worse, they leave a child emotionally stranded and break down the parent-child relationship. These punishments also may result in accidentally *reinforcing* the aggressive behavior.

What to Avoid:
- **Big Reactions:** If we yell, gasp, or dramatically react, even negatively, we may be reinforcing the behavior by providing attention.
- **Using Aggressive Behavior in Return:** One conventional parenting practice is to slap your child's hand when they hit you or to bite your child when they bite you in an effort to demonstrate how it feels to be on the receiving end of this behavior. Please know that this is *neither effective nor safe*. Fear is a poor teacher, and it's never appropriate to physically reprimand a child. We teach by modeling better behavior and teaching skills.
- **Giving In:** If a child hits or bites to get something and we give in to avoid a meltdown, we've taught them that this behavior is effective.
- **Overexplaining:** Toddlers can't process long lectures. Trying to reason extensively after hitting can become more about attention than learning.
- **Physical Restriction:** Physically restricting your child's hand from hitting triggers their fight-or-flight stress response, and they will likely push back even harder.

What to Do Instead:
- **Establish Physical Safety:** Make sure you and your child are

physically safe by disrupting the unsafe behavior. This might look like moving your child or moving away from them.
- **Stay Calm and Neutral:** A simple "Oh! You hit me" delivered with a calm tone is more effective than a loud reaction and gives you time to calm down while creating emotional safety.
- **Create Connection:** Observe and describe what you see to help your child feel seen and heard: "You wanted the scissors, and I wouldn't give them to you."
- **Set Limits:** Following through is just as important as setting the limit. Tell them, "I won't let you hit me. Hitting hurts." Then put your child down and create some space.
- **Teach Skills:** Once your child is calm, focus on helping them learn other ways to communicate their feelings. This takes lots of practice and repetition.
- **Keep It Brief:** Use short, clear messages paired with actions: "Biting hurts. You can bite this toy."

That last point brings me to the power of **redirection**. Redirection is one of the most effective tools in your parenting tool kit because it helps toddlers shift away from an unacceptable behavior *without* making them feel ashamed or punishing them. Think of redirection as changing the channel on a TV—you're guiding your child's attention toward something more positive and productive.

Here's why it works:

- **Interrupts the Behavior:** Redirecting stops the unwanted behavior in its tracks by offering a new focus.
- **Preserves Connection:** Instead of scolding, you're engaging with your child in a supportive way.
- **Teaches Alternatives:** Redirection models acceptable ways to act, helping your toddler learn what *to* do instead.

Examples of Redirection in Action
- **Hitting:** "You can ball your hands into fists like this when you are mad."

- **Throwing:** "Let's throw these balled-up socks into the basket instead!"
- **Biting:** "You can bite this teething toy when you feel like biting."

Redirection doesn't mean ignoring the behavior—it's about offering your child an alternative that meets the same need but in a safer, healthier way. By doing this consistently, you'll see your toddler start to develop better coping strategies over time.

Supporting your child in expressing and processing their emotions in a healthy way—through crying, talking, or even stomping their feet—*while* following through on limits is what creates change. Children need time to learn more complex calming skills and gain life experience. Their brains also need time to develop the impulse control required to manage emotions without acting out.

Remember, new behaviors take time to learn, and your toddler will need *many* opportunities to practice. This is a long-game approach—you've got this!

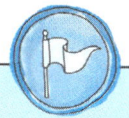

RED FLAG
When to Seek Support

If your toddler's behavior seems to be excessively intense and out of control for longer than a few weeks, and you cannot cope with their behavior on your own, consult your pediatrician. Here are some other warning signs to look out for:
- physical injury to themselves or others (teeth marks, bruises, head injuries)
- regular attacks on you or other adults
- being sent home or barred from play by neighbors or school
- your own fear for the safety of those around them

FAQs

My toddler keeps pulling my hair. What should I do?

Instead of saying, "Ouch! Stop hurting me!" try saying, "Let go of my hair, please. Pulling hair hurts." Keep in mind that when a child does something that causes us pain, we don't want to give them too much power or make them responsible for our feelings and emotions. It's too much for a child to mentally and emotionally handle. Consider offering something else they can tug on, like a soft toy or blanket. They're not being mean—they're exploring, communicating, or looking for connection.

My toddler keeps pushing down other kids. What do I do?

Toddlers push because they're learning how to navigate social situations and looking for ways to exert power, not because they're bad. Step in calmly, say, "I can't let you push," and show them how to ask for a toy or space. Stay close until they learn better ways to communicate.

My toddler laughs after he hits me. Does he think it's funny to hurt me?

Nope. Your toddler is laughing because he feels out of control and is experiencing big emotions like fear and anxiety. This is also true for other out-of-control behaviors. Laughter is one way toddlers release feelings of fear, and it's a sign your child is very dysregulated. It's an automatic reaction to feeling overwhelmed and out of control from having too much power in that moment. Instead of saying things like "Stop laughing!" "This is *not* funny!" or "You hurt Mommy," try, "You hit me, and now you are smiling/laughing." "What are you trying to tell me?" "I wonder if you feel uncomfortable because you bit me."

Chapter 32
OVERCOMING SLEEP CHALLENGES

The clock strikes 8:30 p.m., and you're knee-deep in what can only be described as the "bedtime standoff." Your toddler, wide-eyed and brimming with boundless energy, is running laps around the living room like a miniature marathoner, defying all logic—and the bedtime routine you painstakingly orchestrated. Bath? Check. Books? Check. Snuggles? Double check. And yet, here you are, herding your pint-size insomniac toward the bedroom for the third time tonight.

That's when the negotiations begin: "Just one more story! Pleeeeease, just one more!" Followed by an urgent trip to the bathroom, an even more urgent request for water, and finally, the dreaded battle cry: "I'm not tired!" Let's face it: No one has a longer bedtime to-do list than a toddler. Of course, just when you think you've conquered bedtime, there's a two o'clock wake-up call. Or that reliable afternoon nap suddenly goes off the rails. For many parents, toddler sleep feels like chasing a moving target: elusive, unpredictable, and downright exhausting.

It's in these moments when frustration bubbles over that the doubts creep in. *Why won't they just go to sleep?* You're exhausted. You never knew you'd spend so much time convincing someone *so tired* to go to sleep. You just want to reclaim a sliver of adulthood—a quiet moment to breathe, to think, to feel human—before crashing into bed yourself.

The good news? These sleep challenges aren't signs that you're failing.

They're proof that your toddler's brain is growing, their independence is emerging, and their world is expanding in ways they don't yet understand. The key is learning how to work with these changes rather than fight against them.

Why Won't My Child Sleep?

Sleep, especially for toddlers, is a deeply complex process influenced by their physical needs, emotional state, sensory needs, and developmental milestones. At this stage, your child's brain is growing rapidly, working overtime to process new skills, emotions, and experiences. All this activity can make it harder for them to wind down at the end of the day, even when their bodies are clearly tired.

While sleep disruptions such as waking during the night can be developmentally normal, understanding the *why* behind your child's challenges—whether physical, emotional, sensory, or developmental—you can take steps to address them in a loving and effective way.

Before diving into specific causes, it's important to understand how much sleep your toddler needs. According to the American Academy of Sleep Medicine, toddlers between one and two years old require *eleven to fourteen hours of sleep within a twenty-four-hour period*, including naps. Kids aged three to five need slightly less—*ten to thirteen hours*, including naps.[1]

While these ranges provide a helpful guideline, every child is unique and some kids (like mine) have low sleep needs, meaning they sleep less than the average but are still content and function just fine. If you have to wake your child in the morning, it's a sign they need more sleep and can probably benefit from an earlier bedtime.

Also, it's important to focus not just on the quantity of sleep but also its quality. Sleep isn't just about logging hours; it's about how restorative those hours are. Quality sleep allows your child's brain to grow, process emotions, and recharge for the developmental milestones they're tackling every day. A lack of quality sleep can have a negative impact on your child's behavior, including their attention span, the number of tantrums they are having, and their ability to stay awake—the same as a lack of sleep. So when sleep is disrupted, whether by external factors or internal changes, it can affect their mood, attention span, and behavior.

Physical Causes

Physical discomfort is one of the most common reasons toddlers struggle with sleep. Teething pain, wet diapers, or being too hot or too cold can keep them awake. More subtle issues, such as food sensitivities, eczema, sleep-disordered breathing, or environmental allergens, might also play a role. Add in the challenge of changes in routine—like vacations or adjusting to new time zones—and their tiny systems can easily become overwhelmed. Even their sleep environment can make a big difference. Noise, light, or the texture of their pajamas, which might go unnoticed during the day, can seem magnified at night, making it harder for them to settle. Additionally, it's important to make sure your child has enough sleep pressure built up before bedtime. If your child is unable to fall asleep and bedtime creeps later and later, it might be a sign of a lack of sleep pressure, meaning they are getting too much daytime sleep.

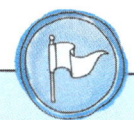

RED FLAG
Sleep-Disordered Breathing (SDB)

One often-overlooked cause of physical sleep challenges is **sleep-disordered breathing (SDB)**. Conditions like enlarged tonsils or adenoids can cause obstructive sleep apnea or chronic snoring, disrupting your toddler's ability to get restorative sleep. If your child frequently snores, mouth breathes, is excessively restless and sweating while sleeping, or wakes up seemingly tired despite a full night's rest, please discuss these symptoms with your pediatrician or an airway dentist.

> For more information, visit transformingtoddlerhood.com/bookresources.

Emotional Causes

Toddlers thrive on connection, and bedtime can feel like an overwhelming separation from the safety of their parents. If your child is waking up in the middle of the night, they may be seeking reassurance and comfort, especially during periods of separation anxiety.

The bedtime routine itself can also play a role. If the evening feels rushed or lacks sufficient connection, your toddler may struggle to transition from the busy world of daytime to the stillness of night. Addressing these emotional needs with a calm, consistent bedtime routine can help foster a sense of security.

Sensory Causes

For toddlers, sensory regulation plays a major role in their ability to calm and fall asleep. Their developing sensory systems sometimes struggle to "power down" after a day filled with stimulation. Additionally, overtiredness, in particular, can cause their bodies to release cortisol, a stress hormone that makes it even harder to relax and fall asleep. By incorporating sensory and calming tools, you can help soothe their nervous system and prepare their body for rest.

Developmental Causes

Just when you think you've nailed your toddler's sleep routine, along comes a sleep regression to throw things off course. These regressions, often hitting around eighteen months, two years, two and a half years, and three years, are normal but frustrating. Regressions are usually tied to big developmental milestones—like language bursts, increased mobility, or the onset of separation anxiety. Your toddler's brain is working overtime, which can make it harder for them to settle down and rest. The key during these periods is to stay consistent. Do your best to stick with your routine (while comforting as needed), which will help them adjust more quickly once the regression passes.

> **TODDLER TIP**
> *Implement a Visual Routine*
>
> Make a visual chart of your child's bedtime routine and hang it up. (If you have an older toddler, get them involved in choosing the routine and creating the chart.) Now, instead of constantly telling your child what to do, they can look at the visual routine and choose what to do next. You get to become a partner in the execution instead of an opposing force telling them what to do.

Preparing Your Child for Sleep

Toddlers are explorers, and their little brains and bodies can be exhausted and overwhelmed by the end of the day, leaving them restless, fidgety, or even wired when they should be winding down. Understanding how to support your toddler's sensory system during bedtime can be a game changer. This also enables you to create a strong emotional connection, which will help your child feel more comfortable separating from you.

By weaving calming sensory tools and connection-rich moments into your bedtime routine, you create an environment that soothes their senses, reduces anxiety, and nurtures their emotional needs. Together, these strategies (along with firm yet respectful limits) turn bedtime from a nightly battle into a time for bonding, reassurance, and rest. Here are some tips that can help you set the stage for a more peaceful and connected bedtime:

- **Experiment with Deep Pressure:** Use a weighted blanket or offer firm squeezes on their limbs and back rubs to help your child feel secure and calm before bed.

- **Check for Comfort:** Choose soft, breathable pajamas and bedding without irritating tags or seams to reduce distractions from sensory discomfort.
- **Create Soothing Sounds:** Use white noise, nature sounds, or soft lullabies to drown out sudden noises and signal to your child's brain that it's time to sleep.
- **Incorporate Calming Scents:** For children over three, add a drop of lavender or chamomile essential oil to a diffuser, bath, or pillow to create a relaxing atmosphere.
- **Use Rhythmic Motion:** Rocking or gentle swinging before bed can help regulate your child's proprioceptive system, preparing their body for rest.
- **Adjust Lighting:** Dim lights an hour before bedtime to mimic natural cues for sleep and, if needed, use a soft nightlight to ease fears of the dark. For some, you may want to ensure that the room is completely dark. Be sure to use blackout shades to block sunlight.
- **Create Rituals:** Before the lights go out, take your child on a "goodnight tour" of their favorite things. Say goodnight to their toys, the stars outside, even the family pet. This ritual builds connection and gives them a sense of closure before they settle down.
- **Use Positive Anticipation:** Reassure your toddler that you're looking forward to seeing them in the morning. Try something like "I can't wait to give you a big hug when you wake up! For now, it's time to rest."
- **Process the Day:** Reflect on the highlights of your child's day during bedtime to provide emotional closure and connection.
- **Simplify Choices:** Offer limited choices like "Would you like to wear the blue pajamas or the red ones?" to give a sense of control.
- **Introduce a Calming Routine:** Follow a predictable sequence of warm bath, massage, story time, and snuggles to signal that sleep is near.
- **Try Gentle Sleep Coaching:** Help your child learn to fall asleep independently with the "gradual retreat" method. Stay with them as they fall asleep, then slowly move farther away each night until they're comfortable sleeping on their own.

- **Be Consistent:** Stick to the routine most nights to help your child feel secure and know what to expect.

These tips combine sensory regulation and connection to create a bedtime routine that soothes your child's nervous system and nurtures emotional security, making sleep a more peaceful process for everyone. You don't have to do them all. Experiment with them and prioritize what works for your family.

Five Common Sleep Challenges

Even with the perfect bedtime routine, sleep challenges often pop up, throwing your plans off course. Toddlers are nothing if not unpredictable, and navigating these hurdles requires patience, consistency, and a little strategy. Here's how to handle the most common issues.

Challenge 1: Bedtime Power Struggles and Tantrums

Bedtime battles are legendary for a reason—toddlers are experts at stalling. One more drink, one more story, one more reason they can't go to sleep. Remember, toddlers crave connection. All the stalling might be a bid for connection or a way of testing limits. Clear, consistent, yet kind limits help them feel safe.

What to Do: Make sure your child's needs are met. Anticipate requests and increase connection to get ahead of the power struggle. If your toddler always asks for water or a snack, be sure they have a snack on time and water in their room. Set limits on the number of books, hugs, and songs. Set the expectation in advance and count them down: "Two more books, then it's time for bed. One more book, then it's time for bed." When they push back or have a tantrum, comfort your child, but remain firm: Bedtime is bedtime. Toddlers learn that when you calmly follow through on limits while still taking their emotional needs into account, they are nonnegotiable—and eventually, the bedtime battles will subside.

Challenge 2: Middle-of-the-Night Wake-Ups

Night wakings can feel endless, especially when you're exhausted, but how you respond is key. While overtiredness, sleep regressions, or a desire for connection often contribute, it's also important to remember that waking during the night is developmentally appropriate for many toddlers. Their brains and bodies are still maturing, and nighttime disruptions are often a normal part of that process.

What to Do: The trick here is not to overreact. First, wait a few moments before rushing to their side to see if your child is actually awake or just shifting between sleep cycles. Resist the temptation to turn the wake-up into a full-blown event, like turning on the lights or getting a snack just to get them back to sleep. Instead, stay calm, offer reassurance, and guide them gently back to bed. Keep the interaction brief and boring, so they understand that nighttime is for sleeping, not for chatting or playtime. If your toddler comes to your room, gently walk them back to bed without much fanfare.

Challenge 3: Early Rising

If your toddler is greeting the day before the sun does, you're not alone. Early rising is a common challenge for many families. Toddlers are notorious for waking up with the first light, eager to start the day, even when you're desperate for just a little more sleep.

What to Do: Children usually need an earlier bedtime, as being overtired can cause middle-of-the-night wake-ups and early rising. Also, utilize blackout shades to keep light out. Consider using a toddler wake-up clock with lights to indicate when it's time to get up. Toddlers love visual cues, and they help reinforce that waking up early doesn't mean starting the day. Only use this tool if you are willing to help your child follow through on the limit. Toddlers won't just automatically listen to the clock in the beginning. Start by setting it when they normally wake up, then push it back by five minutes every few days until you get to at least six o'clock. If early rising persists, adjust your expectations (and set the coffee to brew automatically). You might have a child with low sleep needs.

Challenge 4: Dropping Naps

Transitioning from two naps to one—or from naps to no naps at all—is a major shift. This process typically begins around 12 to 18 months (for two naps to one) and 2.5 to 4 years old (for no naps).

What to Do: Follow your toddler's lead. If they skip naps or resist, shift toward one midday nap or introduce quiet time. During quiet time, offer books, audiobooks, or quiet toys and keep the atmosphere restful. Remember, you can't force your child to take a nap no matter how badly they need one. Toddlers rarely drop a nap all at once. They might only nap every other day before fully dropping a nap. When your toddler does skip a nap, putting them to bed thirty to sixty minutes early can help prevent them from becoming overtired, causing middle-of-the-night and early wake-ups. Additionally, sometimes limiting a nap to an hour is helpful to keep your toddler napping without pushing bedtime too late. When your toddler no longer naps, expect there to be times they struggle to make it to bedtime or fall asleep in the car and consequently stay awake until ten. This stage is challenging yet temporary.

Challenge 5: Transitioning to a Toddler Bed

Moving from a crib to a toddler bed is exciting but often comes with newfound freedom (and limit testing). Most toddlers make this shift between 2.5 and 3.5 years old; however, some kids transition to a Montessori floor bed around 15 months. It's important to ensure a safe sleep environment and practices.

What to Do: Prepare your child by talking about the transition in advance. Set clear expectations: "Once you're in bed, it's time to stay there until your clock says it's okay to get up." Make sure the room is safe and secure by anchoring heavy furniture, covering outlets, securing cords, and removing small or sharp objects. Use a baby gate to keep your child from roaming the house if needed. Keep toys and stimulating items out of reach at bedtime to encourage a calm sleep environment. Use a toddler clock or lamp on a timer to provide visual cues and stay consistent with limits.

By approaching these common sleep challenges with consistency, calmness, and a bit of flexibility, you can manage the bumps along the way without losing your cool (or too much sleep).

Turning Bedtime Challenges into Connection

Your toddler's reluctance to sleep isn't defiance—it's a request for reassurance and assistance. Sleep isn't a one-size-fits-all process, and it changes as your child grows. Some transitions will feel seamless; others might leave you questioning everything. But the goal isn't perfection—it's creating a routine that supports healthy sleep habits, nurtures your child's sense of security, and fosters calm.

Remember, you can't control whether your child falls asleep, but you can provide the environment and tools they need to get there. Stay neutral, stick to your boundaries, and trust the process. Toddlerhood is a journey—and so is sleep. With patience, persistence, and a little flexibility, you'll find your rhythm. And before you know it, bedtime won't be just another challenge—it'll be a cherished part of your day.

FAQs

My child is suddenly afraid of monsters. What should I do?

Sudden fears are common as toddlers' imaginations grow. Avoid reinforcing the fear with "monster spray" or similar tricks, as this can imply monsters are real. Instead, validate your child's feelings: "I know monsters seem scary, and they aren't real." Then calmly check the closet or under the bed together, showing them there's nothing there. Reassure them with grounding statements like "You are safe in our home."

My toddler keeps coming out of their room after bedtime. What should I do?

This is common! Be sure to create lots of connection in the bedtime routine. If your child comes out, gently walk them back to their room without fanfare. It can help to have a consistent phrase to say, such as, "I love you and it's time for bed." Stay consistent to help reinforce the limit. Additionally, you can choose to stay with your child until they fall asleep or try time checks. Come back and check on your toddler before they get out of bed. Give them reassurance and leave, then check in again. Slowly extend the amount of time before you check in—from one minute to three minutes to five minutes and so on. Eventually, your child will feel secure enough to stay in bed.

How do I help my toddler adjust to a new time zone or time change?

You can start adjusting your toddler's schedule a few days before your trip by shifting meals, naps, and bedtime toward the new time zone, or if you have a long international plane ride, start making adjustments at your destination. Once you arrive, expose them to natural light and keep meals and naps on the local schedule. Be patient—it may take a few days for their internal clock to reset. For daylight savings, if your child is an early riser, do nothing—the clock springing forward will work in your favor. If your child is already going to bed too late, then move their schedule fifteen minutes earlier each day three days in advance for bedtime and waking them up. At the end of daylight savings, do the opposite, moving everything fifteen minutes later for three days if your child is going to bed too early. Don't stress! They will eventually adjust, even if it takes a couple of weeks.

What's the difference between nightmares and night terrors?

Nightmares tend to happen later in the night and may wake your child, leaving them scared and needing comfort. Reassure them with calm words and a comforting presence.

Night terrors tend to occur earlier in the night, often causing your child to scream or thrash while still asleep. They usually won't remember the episode. Stay nearby to ensure they are safe, but avoid waking them.

Chapter 33

BRUSHING AND CARING FOR TEETH

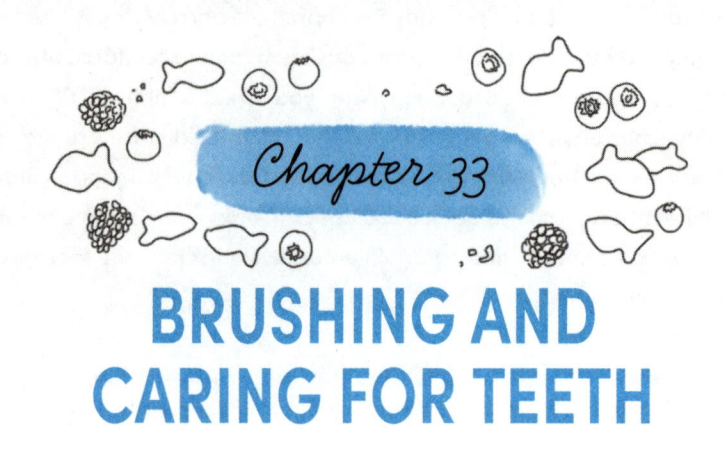

It's the end of a long day, and you just want to get your toddler to brush their teeth before bed. But instead of gleaming smiles, you're met with defiance. They clamp their mouth shut or insist on doing it themself, only to barely graze their teeth with the brush or just eat the toothpaste. Sound familiar? You're not alone.

Toddlers crave independence, especially when it comes to their bodies. They quickly figure out that brushing their teeth is something you can't force, and the more they sense how much you care about it, the more they dig in their heels. It's not about being difficult—it's about learning they have agency. This push-pull is the heart of toddler development: asserting autonomy while navigating limits. Understanding this dynamic can help transform toothbrushing from a nightly power struggle into an opportunity to support their growing independence—while keeping those pearly whites healthy.

What to Do If Your Toddler Resists

If your toddler is resisting, it's tempting to explain the importance of toothbrushing—after all, you want them to understand why it's necessary! But even if you calmly get down on their level and explain that brushing prevents cavities and keeps their breath fresh, chances are they'll still resist.

Why?

Because at that moment, they don't care about cavities; they care about how they're feeling.

This is a great example of how we, as adults, approach situations through our logical lens, shaped by a fully developed brain. We think that explaining the importance of toothbrushing will motivate our toddler—but it goes right past them. They're not in their logical brain; they're in their emotional brain.

At that moment, what they need isn't a dental hygiene lecture but *emotional connection*. By meeting them in their emotions, we disarm the power struggle and start calming their emotional storm. When they feel connected, they're much more likely to cooperate. This is the power of connection: It builds trust, fosters understanding, and makes challenging moments more manageable—for both of you.

So connect with them emotionally first and then acknowledge their feelings, saying, "It seems like you don't want to brush your teeth" or "I hear you saying that you don't want to brush your teeth right now." Then pause. Let them express their frustration and offload their emotions. Hold space for it. This is part of the de-escalation process.

Now it's time to find a way forward. You might say something like "It's important to brush our teeth. How can we make this better?" This simple question invites them into the problem-solving process, shifting the dynamic from "parent vs. child" to "we're in this together." By involving your child in cocreating a solution, you're not only reducing the pressure on yourself to figure it out but also teaching valuable life skills like collaboration, problem-solving, and compromise. Maybe they'll suggest picking a favorite toothbrush, playing a song while brushing, or even letting their stuffed animal "go first."

TODDLER TIP
How to Introduce Toothbrushing

When first introducing toothbrushing to your child, hold them on your hip while you brush your teeth, modeling the skill in a pressure-free way. You can also let them practice by brushing your teeth or a stuffed animal's teeth.

Eight Tips to End Toothbrushing Power Struggles

1. **Remove the Pressure:** Stay as neutral as possible. Be nonchalant. Let them play with water, set their toothbrush beside the sink, and start brushing *your* teeth. Keep the mood light and playful, saying "Ahhh" and opening your mouth wide, without applying any pressure. Toddlers are naturally curious and often want to mimic what you're doing. This side-door approach can be far more effective than a direct, head-on battle.

2. **Give Them a Sense of Control:** Let your child choose their toothbrush or toothpaste. When they feel like they have a say, they're more likely to cooperate. You can also give them control during the brushing process: "It's time to brush our teeth. Would you like to start and then I'll finish, or should I do it quickly by myself?"

3. **Encourage Independence:** Make sure your child can access the sink and their toothbrush using a step stool or toddler tower. When you support your child in feeling capable, you are working with their natural development, and it can create more cooperation as a result.

4. **Get Multiple Toothbrushes:** I find it helpful to have three toothbrushes—one for each of your child's hands and one for you. Then you don't need your child to cooperate with taking turns to have a toothbrush to check their teeth.

5. **Create Predictability with Routines:** The more consistent you are with when and how you brush your toddler's teeth, the less room there is for protest. Toddlers thrive on routine, so making toothbrushing a nonnegotiable part of your daily routine as early as possible is helpful. Know your child and what part of the day they have enough bandwidth to brush their teeth. Exhaustion often leads to more resistance.

6. **Make It Fun:** Turn toothbrushing into a game! Sing a silly song while brushing, or pretend you're looking for a piece of broccoli from dinner stuck in their teeth. Making it playful takes the focus away from the task itself and helps shift their emotional state from resistance to curiosity while creating connection.

7. **Think Outside the Box:** If you need to disrupt a cycle of resistance, try brushing at different times and in different places. For example, brush your child's teeth before their bath instead of right before bed—or even during the bath! You might also try brushing teeth in their bedroom. While brushing by the sink is ideal, if your child associates it with a power struggle, mixing up the location can help ease resistance before transitioning back to the sink. Some children even respond better when they lay their heads in your lap while you brush their teeth from above. This change in perspective can make the process more comfortable and less stressful for both of you.

8. **Keep It Positive and Celebrate Progress:** Do your best to make toothbrushing a positive experience by focusing on progress, not perfection. Notice even the smallest efforts your child makes and celebrate them. Ten seconds of cooperative brushing is far better than three minutes of struggle and frustration. If your child only tolerates a few seconds of brushing initially, that's perfectly fine—build from there. Gradually increase the brushing time as they become more comfortable. Start with brushing once a day if that's all they can handle, and work up to more frequent brushing over time.

If your toddler still refuses, you'll need to decide whether to follow through against their will. As the parent, it's your responsibility to keep them healthy and safe—even when they're protesting. If you choose this route, be prepared for big emotions and strong resistance. It's not ideal, as it can add negativity to the experience, so it's best reserved as a last resort. Remember, it's best to focus on creating and building on small experiences. The key is to meet your child where they are and build on small successes.

Weaning from a Pacifier

Let's talk about pacifiers—a common comfort item for toddlers. While pacifiers can be incredibly soothing in the early months of a baby's life and potentially help prevent sudden infant death syndrome (SIDS), extended use can lead to potential issues such as a high, narrow palate, teeth misalignment, speech delays due to reduced oral-motor development, and even recurring ear infections. If your little one is still using a pacifier at age two or later, it's a good time to start thinking about weaning them off of it.

When it comes to pacifier weaning, I get it—this can feel like a monumental task. The pacifier has been a reliable source of comfort and security, not just for your toddler but for you too. But transitioning away from it doesn't have to be a horrible experience. Here's how you can make the process smoother for both of you in three steps.

Step 1: Limit Use

If your toddler is used to having a pacifier all day, start to limit daytime use. Introduce a comfort object for several weeks before making changes to the pacifier routine. When your child asks for their pacifier, give them both the pacifier and the comfort object together. This helps them start forming a connection with the new comfort item. If your child currently has unlimited access to their pacifier, begin by putting it away when they're not using it and only giving it to them when they ask. This small step introduces a gentle boundary and begins to reshape their relationship with the pacifier.

Once your child is comfortable with this change, establish a firmer limit. For example, you might decide the pacifier is only for sleep times.

Outside of those times, keep the pacifier out of sight—this can help keep it out of mind. Store it in a box on their dresser or another place they can't easily reach. You might also consider removing the pacifier from their mouth once they've fallen asleep and putting it away.

Whatever limits you set, be clear and consistent. Consistency is key to helping your child adjust to the new routine!

Step 2: Prepare

There are many ways to prepare your toddler for saying goodbye to their pacifier. Start a few weeks in advance by reading books about letting go of the paci—this helps plant the idea of transitioning in their mind. Then, set a date. Choosing a Friday night can be helpful since you'll have the weekend to support your child through the adjustment.

Make the countdown fun and visual by using sticky notes: five, four, three . . . until the big day arrives. This creates anticipation while giving your child time to process their feelings. Be ready to offer plenty of validation and reassurance along the way: "I know you don't want to give up your paci. I'm here to help you." The more involved they feel in the process, the smoother the transition will be.

If you seem uncertain or hesitant, your toddler will pick up on that anxiety and may cling to their paci even more. Toddlers are experts at reading our vibes—your confidence can make all the difference.

Step 3: Transition

When the day comes to say goodbye completely, you can simply gather all the pacifiers and get rid of them or use a few creative options. The "Pacifier Fairy" could visit (just like the Tooth Fairy), collecting pacifiers and leaving a small toy. Or you could sew the pacifiers into a stuffed animal so they can still "have" them in a new way.

Expect some big feelings. The pacifier has been their go-to comfort for a long time, so it's natural for them to be upset. Hold space for those emotions and let them know it's okay to feel how they feel. Give lots of loving reassurance. Once you've decided to take the pacifier away, stick with it. Waffling can make the whole process more confusing, drawn-out, and emotionally taxing for everyone involved.

And finally—celebrate! This is a huge milestone for both of you. If you're feeling all kinds of emotions about watching your little one grow out of their pacifier stage, that's completely normal. Parenting is full of these bittersweet moments, but you're doing great.

You've Got This!

The struggles may seem never-ending, but with patience, consistency, and creativity, you can turn this daily task into a more positive experience. By validating your toddler's emotions, offering them choices, and adding some fun, you'll gradually reduce the resistance—and you'll be one step closer to a cavity-free toddler with a shining smile!

FAQs

At what age should I take my child to the dentist for the first time?

The American Academy of Pediatric Dentistry recommends taking your child to the dentist by their first birthday or when their first tooth appears.[1] Early dental visits help acclimate your toddler to the dentist's office, making future visits less stressful. Regular checkups also catch any potential issues early, ensuring your toddler's teeth stay healthy.

At what age should I start flossing my child's teeth?

It's recommended to start flossing your child's teeth as soon as two teeth touch, which typically happens between ages two and three.[2] However, introducing flossing earlier—even before it's absolutely necessary—can be beneficial. This gives your child time to practice and become familiar with the process, making it easier when regular flossing becomes essential.

When should I introduce toothbrushing?

It's best to introduce toothbrushing as early as possible—even as early as three to four months old. Use a silicone finger toothbrush or a silicone toothbrush teether to gently clean your baby's gums and emerging teeth. Starting early helps normalize the routine and makes brushing a familiar part of your child's daily life.

It's not recommended to use an electric toothbrush before the age of three. Stick to a soft-bristled manual toothbrush until they're ready.

Chapter 34

TEACHING TOILET-LEARNING SKILLS

Welcome to the great potty-learning adventure! Yes, you read that right—*learning*, not *training*. Let's reframe the narrative right from the start. When you think about it, *potty training* implies it's something you do *to* a child, like teaching a dog to sit or shake hands. But *potty learning* is a term coined by the Montessori approach that focuses on the journey you embark on *with* your child—a partnership that fosters autonomy, confidence, and trust in their developing body.[1]

Now, here's a key mindset shift: Toddlers are transitioning from being passive bystanders in their bodily functions to active participants in managing them. This is no small feat; it requires skill building, opportunities to practice, and plenty of time. After spending one to three years peeing and pooping in diapers, using the toilet isn't second nature—it's an entirely new world. Our role is to guide them with patience and grace as they step into this new chapter of bodily autonomy. Just like with any learning process, there will be bumps along the way, but we'll navigate them with empathy, encouragement, and, yes, a healthy dose of humor.

How Do I Know When My Child Is Ready?

Every child is unique. While there isn't a magic age when your toddler suddenly "gets it," the ideal window to start preparing and casually introducing potty learning typically falls between eighteen and twenty-four months (also the same period when toddlers begin resisting diaper changes—an early sign they're ready for more control) because toddlers tend to be more naturally curious about their bodies and eager for independence during this stage. For some kids this can be as early as twelve months and for others as late as thirty months. There is some research that shows waiting until after three can make potty learning harder. However, it might not be because you waited. It might be because these kids have constipation issues that complicate the process.[2] On the other hand, there is also some research that shows potty learning *before* the age of two can result in developing voiding dysfunction (difficulty or abnormality in the process of urination) because they are more likely to hold their pee and poop.[3]

The takeaway? Kids don't operate on a one-size-fits-all schedule. The key is in knowing your child and working with them toward the goals.

Here are a few key signs that your child may be ready for toilet learning:

- **Increased Body Awareness and Communication:** If your child starts tugging at their diaper after they've wet themselves, they suddenly want privacy while pooping, or they tell you when they have a soiled diaper, that's a clear sign they're beginning to recognize their body's signals. It's the first step in connecting the dots between the feeling of needing to go and the act of using the toilet.

- **Dry Diapers for Longer Periods:** When your toddler starts staying dry for a couple of hours at a time or even after a nap, it's an indication that they're developing awareness and bladder control.

THE PHYSICAL TODDLER

- **Interest in Toileting:** If your little one is curious about what you're doing when you go to the bathroom, it's a great opportunity to start introducing the concept of potty learning. They might follow you in, ask questions, try to flush the toilet, or show an eagerness to imitate what you're doing. Invite this natural curiosity and use it as a springboard to gently guide them toward their own toilet-learning journey.

Remember, the goal isn't to rush your child or fit them into a predetermined schedule. Readiness looks different for every toddler, and that's okay. Also, your child doesn't need to show all of these signs to be ready—it's also about their level of willingness. Focus on introducing small skills into their routines that build over time and bring you to the desired outcome.

TODDLER TIP
Avoid Exerting Pressure and Control

Always keep in mind urination and bowel movements are one of the few things toddlers have *absolute control* over. The more you try to force, pressure, or shame them, the more likely you are to ignite a power struggle.

Instead of pressuring your toddler by saying "You need to go potty. I know you have to go!" try offering supportive guidance: "The potty is right there. You can go when you're ready." Similarly, avoid inviting a power struggle by asking, "Do you want to go potty?" Most toddlers will instinctively say no to assert independence. Instead, give them a sense of control by offering choices: "It's time to use the potty. Do you want to use the big toilet or the small potty?"

Getting Started

Again, there's no one-size-fits-all method for potty learning, and research backs this up.[4] No matter the method, what matters most is meeting your child where they are developmentally and creating realistic expectations. It's very unlikely your child will have completed their potty learning within three days. Some kids can make immense progress in a few days, but remember: Toilet learning is a process of building skills, and it's not linear—your child may make forward leaps and then take a few steps back. Focus on building skills and keeping the process positive and supportive.

Here's how to get started:

Step 1: Transition Diaper Changes to the Bathroom

Start by changing your toddler's diaper while they're standing up in the bathroom. This simple shift helps them connect toileting with the bathroom environment. I began this with my child at ten months when he started resisting diaper changes while lying down. Instead of using distractions, I tuned in to what he was communicating—and realized he was ready for a change. Set up your bathroom with diapering supplies and a small potty to signal that pottying happens there. This step bridges the gap between "I lie down and get changed" to "I sit and use the potty."

Step 2: Prepare the Environment

Having the right supplies can make the process smoother. The following are some things you might want to have handy:

- a small potty and/or seat reducer with a stool
- a bathroom basket with extra underwear, pants, and socks
- stain remover and fabric cleaner
- a basin for rinsing soiled clothes
- paper towels for quick cleanups

Get your child involved in setting up their potty space. This helps them feel excited and invested in the process.

> For a curated list of my favorite potty-learning tools and books, visit transformingtoddlerhood.com/bookresources.

Step 3: Practice Key Skills

If your toddler can follow basic directions like "Go get your shoes" or "Put away your toy," they're developmentally ready to understand and follow the steps involved in toilet learning, such as pulling up/down pants, sitting on the potty, and washing hands afterward. Practice these skills regularly, offering help as needed, and gradually shift responsibility to your child as they gain confidence.

Step 4: Address Constipation Early

Before diving in, check for signs of constipation. Starting toilet learning while your child is constipated can lead to painful bowel movements and stool withholding, creating unnecessary stress and power struggles. See the section on pooping for more details.

Step 5: Mentally Prepare Yourself

Expect some inconvenience and mess—it's part of the process. Prepare mentally for accidents and cleanups so you're not caught off guard. Staying calm and patient helps create a positive learning environment.

Step 6: Prepare Your Child

Introduce the process through books about potty learning, which can help familiarize them with what to expect. Talk openly about toileting steps, making the experience less intimidating and more engaging.

Addressing all of these is important prior to actively potty learning and will help the process go more quickly. Once they are addressed, choose a day to get started (preferably when you can spend several days at home). Round up all of the diapers and remove them from your home; replace them with underpants. If you are only working on daytime pottying, switch to a pull-up diaper at night. This way you are not tempted to go back to diapers when there are several accidents in the beginning. Some kids do best being diaper- and underwear-free in the beginning. Make sure they have easy access to the potty by keeping it nearby wherever you are. Also, practice making pottying part of the routine. Great times to sit on the potty are first thing in the morning or when getting dressed, after breakfast, before and after a nap, before a bath, and before bed. *Offer*, don't pressure. The more attached you seem to be to your toddler sitting on the potty, the more they will push back. Keep it fun and low pressure.

> **TODDLER TIP**
> *Help Your Child Release*
>
> Help your toddler relax while sitting on the potty by giving them something to hold, like a favorite toy or book, to keep their hands busy and their mind focused. Alternatively, you can try fun relaxation tricks like blowing bubbles or blowing water through a straw in a cup to help them release, playing calming music or an audiobook, or reading them a story to help keep them relaxed.

Managing Accidents

Accidents will happen—sometimes in the middle of the night, sometimes in the middle of the grocery store. While you can't control when they occur, you can control how you respond. Shifting your perspective on accidents is key. Accidents aren't failures—they're simply part of the learning process. Just like learning to walk or talk, toilet learning takes practice, patience, and time—especially at night. Your toddler isn't "bad" for having an accident; they're navigating a new skill. In fact, **reframing "accidents" as "misses"** can be helpful.[5] Your child simply missed getting to the toilet on time—and that's okay. Children learn through experience, so trying to prevent every mishap can create power struggles and rob them of important learning moments.

> ### TODDLER TIP
> *Unlearn the Cycle of Shame*
>
> Our words have a lot of power, and sometimes we unknowingly shame our kids when they have an accident. When your toddler has a miss, instead of saying, "Why did you pee in your pants? You know you should go on the potty," stay calm and neutral: "Oops! Pee goes in the potty. You didn't make it to the potty this time. We'll try again next time. Let's clean this up." This response is short, direct, and free from shame or frustration. It shows your child that making a mess isn't a disaster—it's just part of the learning process.

After a miss, guide your toddler through the cleanup, inviting them to help without making it a punishment. Avoid statements like "Well, you made this mess, so now you have to clean it up!" Instead, model teamwork and encouragement, fostering a sense of shared responsibility.

It's natural to feel frustrated when you're cleaning up yet another mess or doing endless loads of laundry. But remember, your words and actions shape how your child feels about themself. Imagine being met with frustration, disappointment, or even shame every time you made a mistake. You'd feel defeated. Now, imagine being a toddler, still figuring out bodily control. Responding with patience and understanding lifts them up and helps them stay motivated to keep learning.

> ### TODDLER TIP
> *Keeping Beds Dry*
>
> Layer your child's mattress with a waterproof pad and fitted sheet *twice*. When an accident happens at three o'clock in the morning, you can simply remove the top layer and avoid the whole middle-of-the-night laundry situation. The result: fewer tears (yours and theirs).

Pooping on the Potty

Potty learning can be tricky, but pooping on the potty often presents the biggest hurdle. Many toddlers struggle with stool withholding, a common issue that can be rooted in physical, emotional, or sensory challenges. Research shows that up to 30 percent of children experience constipation,[6] which can cause painful bowel movements, leading to stool withholding—a cycle that's hard to break. The good news is, with the right approach, you can support your child in feeling more comfortable and confident about using the potty.

It's important to understand why some toddlers have trouble pooping on the potty. The following are some of the many reasons why stool withholding happens:

- **Constipation:** Hard, painful bowel movements can make kids avoid pooping altogether.
- **Sensory Processing Challenges:** Kids with sensory sensitivities or autism may struggle with the sensations associated with pooping.
- **Fear of the Potty:** Some children are afraid they might "fall in," or they might be startled by the sound of poop hitting the water.

- **Anxiety and Control:** Potty learning can feel like a loss of control. Refusing to poop becomes a way for toddlers to assert independence.

Since painful bowel movements are often the root of the problem, keeping your child's stool soft is crucial while also striving to understand your unique child's feelings, emotions, and needs.

Practical Ways to Encourage Pooping on the Potty

- **Stay Calm and Positive:** Approach potty learning with patience and a positive attitude. If your child shows signs they need to poop, gently guide them to the potty.
- **Handle Accidents Without Shame:** If your child poops in their diaper, avoid showing frustration or disappointment. Instead, calmly take the poop to the toilet and say, "Poop goes in the potty." This reinforces where poop belongs without blame or shame.
- **Create a Relaxing Environment:** Keep potty time light and encouraging. Sing songs, read books, or play calming music to help your child relax and stay comfortable while sitting on the potty.
- **Focus on Stool Softening:** Ensure your child's stool stays soft enough to pass easily, reducing the likelihood of withholding. Offer plenty of fluids, fiber-rich foods, pre- and probiotics, and healthy fats like avocado and coconut oil. If needed, consult your pediatrician for additional support.
- **Remove the Pressure:** If potty learning becomes stressful or your child resists, take a break for about four weeks and try again later. Sometimes stepping back helps reset the experience.
- **Respect Their Need for Privacy:** Many children feel more comfortable pooping when they have privacy. Allow them to sit on the potty while you stand a few feet away, offering reassurance without hovering.
- **Model and Narrate the Behavior:** Normalize pooping by leaving the bathroom door open when you go (if appropriate) and narrating the process calmly: "I'm going potty. My body is getting rid of what it doesn't need." Seeing you use the toilet can make the process seem less intimidating.

- **Read Books About Pooping:** Children's books about potty learning can make the experience more familiar and fun. Look for stories featuring characters overcoming potty fears or learning to use the toilet with confidence.
- **Use Positive Language About Poop:** Using negative words like *gross*, *smelly*, or *dirty* can create shame and embarrassment, making potty learning harder. Use the following neutral or positive language instead:
  - "Poop is how our body stays healthy."
  - "Everybody poops—it's part of life!"
  - "You listened to your body!"

By staying supportive, patient, and consistent, you'll help your child feel capable and confident on their potty-learning journey.

Naptime and Overnight

Potty learning doesn't stop when the sun goes down or when you're out and about. Naptime, overnight dryness, and pottying on the go can feel like new frontiers—but they don't have to be overwhelming. With a bit of preparation, a growth mindset, and a lot of patience, you can support your child through these next stages with confidence.

Naptime

Incorporating using the potty before naps as part of your child's daily routine is a simple step that can make a big difference. When it comes to naptime protection, here are some of your options:

- **Diaper:** Great for younger toddlers or those still learning bladder control.
- **Waterproof Diaper Cover Over Underwear:** A good in-between option to contain messes while keeping the sensation of wetness.
- **No Diaper at All:** Best for older toddlers showing consistent daytime dryness.

Consider Developmental Readiness
- **Under Age Two:** Most toddlers under two need extra time for bladder development and may benefit from a diaper during naps.
- **Age Three and Up:** Bladder maturity kicks in around age three, making it a good time to experiment with ditching the nap diaper if your child is staying dry regularly.

> **TODDLER TIP**
> *Make Naptime Easy*
>
> If you go diaper-free during naps, consider moving your child out of the crib so they can get to the potty independently. Place a small potty on a waterproof mat near their bed for easy access and fewer disruptions.

Overnight

Staying dry overnight is a developmental milestone that happens when your child's body is ready. It's influenced by both physical development and learned behavior.

Physical Factors
- **ADH Hormone Production:** The body produces **antidiuretic hormone (ADH)**, which slows urine production at night. Children produce more ADH as they get older, reducing the need to pee while they sleep.
- **Bladder Control:** As kids' bladders mature, they can hold more urine, consolidate output, and stay dry for longer periods.
- **Deep Sleeping:** Children who sleep very deeply may take longer to stay dry at night.

- **Developmental Delays:** Kids with developmental challenges might also need more time.
- **Sleep-Disordered Breathing:** Conditions like mouth breathing and sleep apnea can impact nighttime dryness. (See chapter 32, "Overcoming Sleep Challenges," for more information.)

Overnight potty learning is usually the last stage of toilet learning. Some parents tackle it during daytime potty learning, while others wait until daytime dryness is consistent. There's no exact age when kids need to stop using diapers at night, but most children stay dry between ages four and five.

Many experts suggest starting nighttime potty learning when your child **wakes up dry** in the morning. However, this isn't always a reliable indicator, as some children stay dry overnight but pee in their diaper **as soon as they wake up**.

The earlier you start nighttime potty learning, the sooner your child will likely stay dry. On the flip side, prolonged diaper use at night may delay nighttime potty learning and increase the chances of accidents.

Here are five tips to help you with nighttime potty learning:

1. **Try Bottomless Sleep:** Let your child sleep without bottoms or in easy-to-pull-down pajamas.
2. **Be Prepared:** Keep a small potty, extra pajamas, a laundry hamper, and a nightlight near the bed for quick access.
3. **Limit Fluids:** Reduce drinks an hour before bedtime.
4. **Take Double Potty Trips:** Have your child use the potty *twice* thirty to forty-five minutes before bed.
5. **Do a "Dream Pee":** Before you go to bed, gently wake your child, guide them to the potty, and tuck them back in. This can help reinforce the brain-bladder connection.

By staying patient, prepared, and supportive, you can help your child build confidence and master nighttime potty learning—at their own pace.

THE PHYSICAL TODDLER

> **TODDLER TIP**
> *How to Potty on the Go*
>
> Never put anything between your child and the car seat to protect it unless it came with your car seat or is an approved accessory by your car seat manufacturer, as it could reduce your child's safety in the event of a car accident. Instead, put a waterproof diaper cover on top of underwear to prevent messes in the car seat. I prefer this to a pull-up, which prevents children from feeling when they are wet; a pull-up diaper is essentially a diaper! Constantly switching between underwear and pull-up diapers can create confusion and prolong potty learning.

Toilet learning isn't something that happens overnight, and it isn't a one-size-fits-all experience. The best thing you can do is partner with your toddler, supporting them with love and patience. Celebrate their wins, keep your cool when they stumble, and remember: You're teaching them one of the most basic, yet most important, life skills.

FAQs

My toddler is afraid of public restrooms. What can I do?
Public restrooms can be intimidating due to loud automatic hand dryers and unexpected flushing. To ease your child's fear, place a sticker or sticky note over the automatic flush sensor to prevent sudden flushing. (Just remember to remove it afterward.) If your child is sensitive to noise, consider bringing noise-reducing earmuffs/headphones. Practice visiting public restrooms when your child doesn't need to go, making the experience less stressful and more familiar over time. Alternatively, keep a small kit in your car with a travel potty, small muslin blanket (for privacy), spare

clothes, paper towels, and plastic bags. You can put the portable potty in the back of your car or SUV with a plastic bag liner if a public restroom is too overwhelming or gross to use.

Should I reward my child for using the potty?

Rewards are generally not recommended for potty learning because they rely on external motivation, which can take away from your child's inner sense of accomplishment. Focusing solely on rewards can lead to escalating demands, where your child expects bigger prizes or stops cooperating when rewards aren't offered. If you choose to use rewards, avoid using food as an incentive, and gradually increase the required number of potty successes before earning a reward. However, it's often more effective to partner with your child, offer encouragement, and set realistic expectations based on their development and temperament.

What should I do if my child is regressing?

Regressions are common and often happen when a child experiences a major life change or a stressful event, such as moving, starting daycare, or welcoming a new sibling. Most regressions are temporary and can be managed with patience, support, and consistent routines. If the regression lasts longer than a few weeks or becomes severe, consider talking to your child's pediatrician, as it could indicate an underlying issue.

I want to try standing diaper changes, but how do I manage poop?

Standing diaper changes can be manageable with the right techniques. Have your child bend forward in a "downward dog" pose so you can easily wipe their bottom. Another option is to have your child sit on the potty, lean forward, and hug their knees while you wipe. Both positions make cleanup easier while reinforcing potty use as a natural part of the routine.

Is potty learning really harder for boys than it is for girls?

Research shows there may be some truth to this common belief. On average, girls learn how to use the potty about two to three months earlier than boys, with girls completing potty learning around 32.5 months compared to 35 months for boys. Girls also tend to show readiness signs around 24 months, while boys typically show them closer to 26 months. While these differences are averages, every child is unique, and individual readiness matters more than gender-based expectations.[7]

Chapter 35

ENDING MEALTIME CHAOS

The table is set, hands are washed, and you're ready for a peaceful family meal. But before you can even sit down, your toddler spots their plate and the protest begins—"Eww! I don't like peas!"

You feel the words forming—"This is what I made, so you're eating it!"—but pause for a moment. Do you really want a dinner table standoff where peas become flying missiles? Probably not. Besides, it's far more useful to figure out why peas have suddenly become public enemy number one than to wage war over vegetables.

Maybe there's more to your toddler's rejection than meets the eye. What if refusing peas isn't about the peas at all? Picky eating is rarely about the food itself—it's about autonomy, genetics, sensory preferences, and even environmental factors, such as exposure in utero,[1] and our reactions to our toddlers' shenanigans. Understanding what's driving your toddler's resistance can help you respond with patience and insight, instead of falling into the trap of power struggles. Imagine a stress-free mealtime where you're not counting bites or issuing ultimatums, where connection takes precedence over control. Sounds dreamy, right? Let's explore how to make it a reality.

Setting Realistic Expectations and Knowing Your Role

As toddlers explore their budding autonomy, food often becomes the stage where they assert control. Plus, it's common for toddlers to experience neophobia with food at some point in their development. Saying no to vegetables or refusing a once-favorite food isn't just about being difficult—it's about exercising power over one of the few things they can control: their bodies. This is where the battle for bodily autonomy meets the dinner table, making picky eating and power struggles common milestones in toddler development.

The key to reducing mealtime battles and picky eating is setting realistic expectations, knowing your role—and staying in your lane. It's not your job to control your child. You cannot make your child chew food and swallow it. They are in charge of their own body. As the parent, your job is to provide balanced, nutritious meals and create a positive, low-pressure environment. Your toddler's job is to decide *whether* they want to eat, *what* they'll eat from what's offered, and *how much* they'll consume. If they refuse altogether, that's okay—it's not a reflection of your effort or your parenting. It's simply part of their developmental process.

Your Job	Your Toddler's Job
Offer balanced food options that provide a variety of nutrients.	Choose whether or not to eat at each mealtime.
Create connection by making mealtimes enjoyable.	Decide how much food to eat based on their hunger.
Offer meals and snacks throughout the day at consistent intervals.	Select what to eat from the foods you've provided.

When mealtimes become a struggle, it's often because we've blurred the lines between these roles. We might take it personally if our child doesn't eat the food we've prepared, or we may try to pressure them into "just one more bite" because we are afraid they aren't eating enough.

When you trust this division of responsibility, mealtime becomes less about forcing bites and more about creating an environment where your child can explore food at their own pace. This shift helps reduce power struggles, promotes a healthier relationship with food, and frees you from feeling like you need to micromanage every meal. The goal isn't to make them eat—

it's to give them the space to learn how to listen to their bodies, try new things, and develop lifelong eating habits rooted in choice, not coercion.

> ### SCRIPTS FOR COMMUNICATION
> *Promoting a Healthy Relationship with Food*
>
> Mealtimes are an opportunity to teach your child to listen to their body. You can accomplish this by removing pressure and bribes involving dessert.
>
> | *Avoid Saying* | *Try Saying* |
> |---|---|
> | "Finish your dinner!" | "Do you feel full?" |
> | "You can have dessert if you take three more bites." | "Let's enjoy dessert together." |
> | "You can get down after you eat your broccoli." | "Listen to your body to know when you feel full." |
>
> Asking your child to try an arbitrary number of bites might "work" for some kids, but at what expense? It puts unnecessary pressure on them that can lead to a power struggle with strong-willed kids and people-pleasing in more docile kids. Instead, invite your child to try a bite or even lick a food without requiring a specific number of bites. Remember everyone's role.

Picky Eating

Picky eating tends to show up between ages two and four, and while most kids eventually outgrow it, for some, picky eating can stick around well into childhood—or even adulthood. And if your child has sensory processing challenges or developmental delays, navigating mealtime can be even trickier due to heightened sensitivities to textures, tastes, and smells.

Here's the deal: How you respond as a parent can either ease the struggle or lock picky eating into place. Studies show that pressuring kids to eat—or bribing, begging, or forcing them to try new foods—often backfires, increasing food refusal and picky eating habits.[2]

SCRIPTS FOR COMMUNICATION
Responding to Picky Eating

Scenario
Your toddler says: "Yuck! I don't like this food!"

Avoid Saying
"You get what you get, and you don't get upset."
"Stop being so picky!"

Try Saying
"What can we add to make it better?"
"I hear you, and this is what we are eating for dinner. You don't have to like it."
"That's a new taste."
"You're still learning to like that taste."
"Tell me more."

The key to navigating picky eating is exposure—repeated exposure to new foods over many meals. This will not be a linear adventure. Even touching the food or licking it can be a win. Just because they refused broccoli today doesn't mean next week they won't surprise you by devouring it. Stay patient, stay consistent, and keep the pressure low. Here are my favorite strategies for diffusing picky eating and expanding your child's palate:

- **Offer New Foods Repeatedly:** It may take twelve to seventeen exposures before a toddler accepts a new food.[3] Don't give up after one refusal. "Maybe next time your taste buds will love it!"
- **Prepare Foods Differently:** Your child may love raw carrots but hate steamed ones. Mix it up!
- **Always Serve Something Familiar:** Including at least one food they love on their plate ensures they will eat something and keeps the experience more positive.
- **Get Your Child Involved:** Toddlers love feeling like they have a say. Let them help choose what's for dinner within your boundaries. Ask, "Which vegetables should we put on the menu this week?" Or take your child to the grocery store and let them choose a vegetable to try. Get them involved in meal prep.
- **Stay Neutral:** Avoid reacting emotionally to their rejection. Act like nothing's wrong. The calmer you stay, the better. Don't give it much attention and keep exposing your child to the food.
- **Don't Make Food a Battle:** Remember, your job is to offer food, and their job is to decide whether or not to eat and how much to eat. Avoid pressuring your child.
- **Respect Their Body:** Just like adults, toddlers know when they're hungry and when they're full. Trust them to regulate their own intake.
- **Model the Behavior:** Model eating new foods or trying foods you don't love. Eat the foods you want your child to eat.
- **Serve the Same Meal:** Serve the same meal for the entire family if possible. Letting your child sit on your lap or eat from your plate can create a lot of forward progress.
- **Make It More Appealing:** Sometimes a light seasoning or adding another familiar ingredient from the table can turn a "yuck" into a "yum." A sprinkle of salt, a little butter, a dipping sauce, or maybe even some sprinkles might be all it takes to flip the script.
- **Make It Fun:** Cut food into fun shapes. Get fun utensils, like a food pick or toddler chopsticks, or fun plates.
- **Encourage Exploration:** Let your toddler touch their food with their hands or encourage them to lick it. Kids will learn to eat with

utensils soon enough. If your child is picky, the more exploration, the better. Point out the shape, color, or texture. "Look how green these peas are—like little marbles!"

> **TODDLER TIP**
> *Serve Vegetables First*
>
> Serve your toddler vegetables before dinner to increase their vegetable intake. Research shows this could increase vegetable consumption.[4]

Let go of the pressure to monitor every bite. Remember, eating is more about what your child consumes over several days than at one sitting. Instead, focus on creating a positive mealtime environment. This takes practice, but over time, your toddler will learn to listen to their body and regulate their own eating habits—without any need for battles at the dinner table.

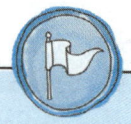

> **RED FLAG**
> *Food Challenges*
>
> If your toddler eats only five to ten foods, is losing weight due to food refusal, only eats food of one color, struggles moving between foods of different textures, has difficulty chewing and swallowing, or gags and chokes on foods, it's important to talk to your pediatrician, as your child may need to work with a feeding therapist to overcome these challenges and expand their ability to eat new foods.

Navigating Food Throwing

Raise your hand if your toddler has ever turned dinner into a projectile experiment. Spaghetti on the walls, Cheerios crushed into the carpet, yogurt dripping off the side of the high chair—you name it, we've all been there. While it can feel personal (*I just made that!*), food throwing is rarely about rejecting your cooking. Instead, it's often a direct expression of play, exploration, and curiosity.

Why Toddlers Throw Food (Hint: It's Not to Annoy You)
- **Play and Exploration:** Dropping spaghetti is classic **trajectory play schema** behavior. They're learning that what goes up (or out) must come down—and watching it happen is endlessly fascinating.
- **Not Hungry:** If your toddler starts tossing food, they may simply be *done eating*. They've reached their fullness cues, and food is now just another sensory material to explore.
- **Feeding a Pet:** Sharing food—even with the family pet—is a toddler's way of practicing caregiving and generosity, and it's also fun! If this is the case, keep your pet in another room during mealtimes.
- **Seeking Connection:** Tossing food can also be a bid for attention: "Look what I can do!" Even a negative reaction can be exciting for a toddler seeking interaction.
- **Dislikes the Food:** Yep, sometimes they just don't like it—but even that's a form of learning! They're figuring out personal preferences and asserting independence.

How to Respond Without Escalating the Situation
- **Start Small:** To minimize the likelihood of food throwing, begin by offering small portions. By giving them a few bites at a time, you not only reduce waste but also make the experience more manageable for their small appetites and attention spans.
- **Stay Calm and Neutral:** The moment you react—whether with frustration or laughter—you've unintentionally made it into a game. I wouldn't give the behavior much attention. You might

even give it zero attention unless it's happened multiple times. If they see that throwing food gets a big reaction, they're more likely to do it again. When food goes flying, calmly say, "You threw your food on the floor. I wonder if you are done eating." This neutral response helps set a boundary without escalating the situation.

- **Don't Rush to Clean Up:** After the food hits the floor, resist the urge to rush and clean it up immediately. Toddlers love cause and effect, and if they throw food and you immediately scramble to clean it up, they might think, *This is fun! I throw, you clean.* Instead, wait until the meal is over to tidy up, or better yet, involve your toddler in the process. Give them a small towel or a broom and let them help with the cleanup. This shows that throwing food has a consequence—they'll have to help clean up the mess—without turning it into a power struggle.

- **Redirect and Reset:** If your toddler continues throwing food, you can gently guide them back to appropriate mealtime behavior. Say something like, "Food stays on your plate. If you don't want it, you can leave it on the side like this." Then model what to do.

- **Set Limits and Follow Through:** If the food throwing persists and they're clearly not interested in eating, it's okay to remove the food for a few minutes. Say something like, "You keep throwing food, so I wonder if you're not hungry right now. You can take a break and come back to it later." Sometimes a short break is all they need to reset their focus and appetite. You might need to set a clear limit and follow through by saying, "I won't let you keep throwing food. I'm going to put you down. You can come back when you are ready to eat," then take them out of their high chair.

When your child does keep their food on their plate, don't forget to give positive attention and acknowledge them: "You kept your food on your plate. Thanks!" Remember, food throwing is a phase, and like all phases in toddlerhood, it will pass. By staying consistent and calm, you're teaching your toddler important lessons about boundaries, self-control, and how to navigate their world.

Getting Them Involved in the Kitchen

Getting your toddler involved in the kitchen is one of the best ways to transform mealtime resistance and picky eating into an opportunity for learning, connection, and fun. It not only makes them feel capable but also gives your child exposure to foods in various forms, which can reduce picky eating. By giving them age-appropriate tasks, you're nurturing your child's developmental need to feel capable and have a role in the family. Plus, kids often become more curious about the foods they're preparing.

Here are some fun, simple tasks for toddlers:

- measuring and pouring ingredients
- assembling small fruit or veggie kebabs
- mixing or stirring ingredients
- setting the table (you can draw a sample place mat for them to follow)
- peeling boiled eggs or tangerines
- mashing soft foods like avocados or potatoes
- cleaning the dishes (kids love soap and water!)
- filling muffin tins or small dishes
- spreading butter or jam

The key to navigating mealtime with toddlers is persistence, flexibility, and patience. Remember, it's completely normal for your child to have lots of wants, needs, and requests while eating. And it's also okay for *you* to stay seated, eat your meal, and respond to their needs when you're ready. With time, consistency, and understanding, you'll build healthier, happier mealtime habits that work for your whole family.

FAQs

It feels like my child is addicted to sugar. How do I reduce their consumption?

Reducing added sugar can have health benefits for your child. The

American Academy of Pediatrics recommends *no added sugar* before age two and *less than twenty-five grams per day* after that.[5] But don't *demonize* sugar. Labeling certain foods as "bad" or banning them completely can trigger power struggles and increase your child's desire for those foods. Instead, avoid bringing foods into your home that you're not comfortable with your child eating. Stock up on snacks they can have unlimited access to.

Need a strategy for weaning off sugary favorites? Try making small swaps. For example, if your child loves store-bought strawberry yogurt with added sugar, try making your own with fresh or frozen strawberries, adding a touch of honey if needed. Or mix plain yogurt into their favorite sugary brand, gradually increasing the plain yogurt ratio over time.

My toddler refuses to eat dinner. What do I do?

First, know that this is *super* common. Toddlers are naturally inconsistent eaters, so try not to stress if dinner gets skipped. Make sure your child isn't filling up on milk and snacks right before a meal to ensure they come to the table hungry. If your child refuses to eat dinner and you know there is at least one thing on their plate that they will eat, then put the dinner aside. When they ask for a snack or say they are hungry a bit later, reoffer them their dinner. Sometimes kids refuse dinner because they are looking forward to their bedtime snack. An alternative is to serve a boring bedtime snack. You don't want snacks to be more exciting than meals. Stay calm, avoid power struggles, and trust that your child will eat when they're hungry.

My toddler won't sit at the table. They keep running off. What should I do?

Your toddler's attention span is short, so expecting them to sit at the table for an extended period is unrealistic. Set them up for success by seating them at the table *with* their food, not before. Make mealtime engaging—play soft dinner music, dim the lights, and include them in the conversation. Flexibility is key. Some nights, your child may need to leave and return to the table later. I've had nights where my child needed to move, so I placed their plate on a stool beside the table, allowing them to play between bites. The ability to sit for longer periods will come with practice and brain maturity. (Check out chapter 13, "Setting Realistic Expectations," for more.)

How do I help my child develop a healthy relationship with food?

From the moment they're born, babies instinctively listen to their bodies. They know when they're hungry, when they're full, and what they need. Our job as parents is to nurture that inner wisdom—not drown it out with our worry about whether they've eaten enough peas or gotten enough protein.

Take the pressure out of mealtime. Avoid labeling foods as "good" or "bad," and don't talk about dieting, weight, or body image around your child. Keep meals positive and never use food as a reward or punishment. Offering a wide variety of foods regularly helps kids learn balance naturally. Explain the difference between hunger and fullness and encourage your child to listen to their body, without pressuring them to eat more. Additionally, avoid holding dessert hostage. Instead, serve dessert alongside dinner occasionally—it removes the "forbidden fruit" appeal and teaches kids that all foods fit.

Chapter 36

BALANCING SAFETY AND EXPLORATION

You're watching your little one walk across a log at the park, their little arms outstretched for balance, and suddenly you feel that familiar knot in your stomach—the one that screams *Danger!* Without thinking, those two words leap from your mouth: "Be careful!" It feels like protection, a reflex designed to shield them from any potential threat. But more often than not, "Be careful!" is a vague reaction to your own fear rather than a true warning of danger. It doesn't give your child the specific feedback and tools they need to understand the risk and navigate it, and, worse yet, it can dim their spark of curiosity and adventurous spirit when overused.

Toddlers are natural explorers. They're wired to seek out new challenges, to push the limits of their bodies, and to test the boundaries of their world. They climb trees, scale playgrounds, and balance on curbs—not because they want to terrify you but because they're learning. They're figuring out how their bodies move, how gravity works, and how to solve problems. And yes, it's your job as a parent to keep your child safe. It can be tempting to want to plaster your child in Bubble Wrap every step of the way. But research shows risky play—like roughhousing, climbing, or balancing—is not just a phase that toddlers go through; it's essential for their development. It builds self-confidence, resilience, and problem-solving skills.[1] They learn how far they can push themselves, how to get out of sticky situations, and how to bounce back from mistakes.

TYPES OF RISKY PLAY FOR TODDLERS

Below are some types of risky play that are essential for toddlers' growth and development. While these activities help children explore their limits and build new skills, they come with inherent challenges and should always be supervised to ensure a safe, supportive environment.

Playing at Height
- climbing trees, jungle gyms, or rock walls
- walking along balance beams or logs
- jumping from low platforms or rocks

Playing with Speed
- riding scooters, tricycles, or balance bikes fast
- running downhill or across uneven terrain
- sledding down gentle slopes
- racing with friends or family

Play Involving Tools
- digging with child-safe gardening tools
- cutting fruit with toddler-safe knives
- cutting paper with toddler-safe scissors

Play Involving Potentially Dangerous Elements
- splashing and wading in shallow water (with adult supervision)
- roasting marshmallows near a campfire
- candlelit dinners or blowing out birthday candles
- mud play with water hoses or small sprinklers

Roughhousing or Rough-and-Tumble Play
- play wrestling with siblings or friends
- pillow fights or mock sword fighting with foam sticks
- rolling around on soft mats or grassy areas
- tug-of-war with ropes or fabric strips

Play with Risk for Disappearing or Getting Lost
- playing hide-and-seek
- exploring neighborhood trails or familiar hiking paths
- creating "adventure" games in enclosed play areas
- building forts and dens in the backyard or playroom

Play Involving Impacts
- crashing into foam blocks or soft objects
- bumper car–style games with ride-on toys
- jumping into piles of leaves or snow
- running and bouncing off padded walls in play centers

So the next time you feel that instinct to shout "Be careful!" bubbling up, take a breath and ask yourself: *Are they in actual danger, or am I just feeling nervous?* If there's real risk—like your child is about to touch a hot stove or run into the street—then it's time to use clear, direct language like "Stop!" or "Freeze!" These words are sharp and specific; they cut through the moment and get your child's attention fast.

But if your child is simply navigating a new challenge, try swapping "Be careful" for a more intentional approach. Engage with curiosity, offer specific guidance, and help your child build awareness. Rather than calling out a vague warning, give your toddler something they can work with, something that helps them tune in to their body and the environment around them.

Instead of "Be careful!" try approaching risky situations from one of these angles:

- **Curiosity:** "What's your plan?"
- **Guidance:** "Focus on your feet."
- **Problem-Solving:** "How will you go up or go down?"
- **Creating Awareness:** "Do you hear the cars? The road is close."

For example: When your child is climbing, resist the urge to hover. Watch how they navigate the challenge. Are they struggling to find their footing? Offer a calm, specific prompt like "What can you find to hold on to?" or "What do you need to do next?" These questions guide them toward their own solutions, fostering independence and self-reliance. They invite your child to think critically about the situation so they can navigate it safely.

Children will gain problem-solving skills and build confidence as they learn to assess and manage challenges on their own. And while risky play is important, so is making your home a safe space for exploration. Secure furniture with wall anchors, cover outlets, remove choking hazards, and teach safety around hot drinks and sharp objects. When your home is toddler-proofed, you can relax more and let your child explore with confidence.

Here's the takeaway: It's not about eliminating risk but managing it. Your job is to create an environment where your child can safely test their limits. This means supervising risky play—being close enough to step in if needed but far enough to let them problem-solve independently.

SCRIPTS FOR COMMUNICATION
Unlearning Shame

When your child tests a limit and gets a scrape or a bump, it's important to remember they are not being bad—they are experimenting and exploring in a developmentally appropriate way.

> Avoid using shame or blame, which can make them less likely to take healthy risks in the future. Instead, start with connection by offering reassurance to soothe them. Then you can follow up by restating limits and teaching skills as needed to keep your child safe.
>
> **Avoid Saying:** "How many times do I have to tell you not to do that?"
> **Try Saying:** "Are you okay? That must hurt."
>
> **Avoid Saying:** "I told you not to run."
> **Try Saying:** "Mommy's here. It's okay."

Roughhousing

Now, let's talk about another form of play that might send your heart racing: roughhousing. Think wrestling on the floor, tumbling over couches, pillow fights, chasing, or play fighting. It can look chaotic, loud, and maybe even a little risky—but there's more to it than meets the eye.

> **Myth:** Roughhousing makes toddlers aggressive, condones fighting, and leads to injuries.
> **Fact:** Rough-and-tumble play is a powerful tool for child development.

Bottom line: This kind of play is *good* for your toddler.

Research shows that rough-and-tumble play builds physical strength, coordination, and spatial awareness.[2] And it goes beyond just the physical—it's also key to emotional and social growth. Kids who engage in this type of play tend to be better at regulating their emotions, managing frustration, and understanding social cues. It teaches them boundaries and empathy, as they learn how to play without hurting others and adjust their behavior when things get too intense.

Roughhousing is also a prime opportunity to practice consent. When toddlers roughhouse with adults, they benefit from having a guide who can model emotional regulation, set and reinforce boundaries, and give words to actions and feelings. Setting limits isn't about shutting down the fun—it's about helping toddlers learn how far they can take roughhousing and recognizing when it's time to pause or change the game. When things get too intense, you can step in with compassion and guidance, teaching them how to read social cues, use their words, and navigate physical interactions with care. So next time a pillow fight breaks out, know that you're not just playing—you're building lifelong skills.

Creating a safe environment doesn't mean shielding your child from every risk—it means giving them the freedom to explore while managing potential dangers. With thoughtful supervision and a well-prepared space, you'll help your child build confidence, independence, and the skills they need to navigate the world safely.

TODDLER TIP
Always Wear Helmets

Safety first, fun always! Helmets should be a *must* anytime your toddler hops on a bike, scooter, or skateboard. Choose a well-fitted helmet that stays securely in place—no wobbling allowed. Make it part of the adventure by modeling helmet-wearing yourself and letting your toddler pick out a fun design they love.

FAQs

Roughhousing between my kids starts out fine, but it gets out of control, and everyone ends up in tears. How do I prevent this from happening?

Since toddlers have limited impulse control, roughhousing can escalate quickly. Adult supervision helps keep play fun and safe. Stay nearby so you can step in before things get out of control. Regularly check in with each child by asking, "Are you both still having fun?" or "Does anyone need a break?" If tears happen, avoid shaming. Comfort both kids, ensure everyone is okay, and guide them in making amends. (See chapter 42, "Managing Sibling Conflict," for more detailed strategies.)

I want to take my toddler swimming but also have an infant. How do I keep everyone safe?

This can be tricky, as toddlers and infants have very different needs. Whenever possible, aim for an even adult-to-child ratio. If you're on your own, make sure both kids are in coast guard–approved life jackets and stay within arm's reach at all times. Consider visiting a pool with lifeguards or bringing a trusted adult to help supervise. Also, make sure your kids' swimsuits are brightly colored so they can be seen if they go underwater. Blue, white, beige, and green suits are the hardest to see when a child is submerged.

Does roughhousing make kids aggressive?

No, research shows that roughhousing actually helps kids develop self-control, emotional regulation, and positive social skills. However, kids can get carried away, so it's essential for adults to supervise and step in before someone gets hurt. Roughhousing with an adult also provides opportunities to practice consent and self-control, as adults can model these skills and introduce pauses to teach healthy boundaries. Both boys and girls benefit from rough-and-tumble play.[3]

Chapter 37

PLAYING INDEPENDENTLY

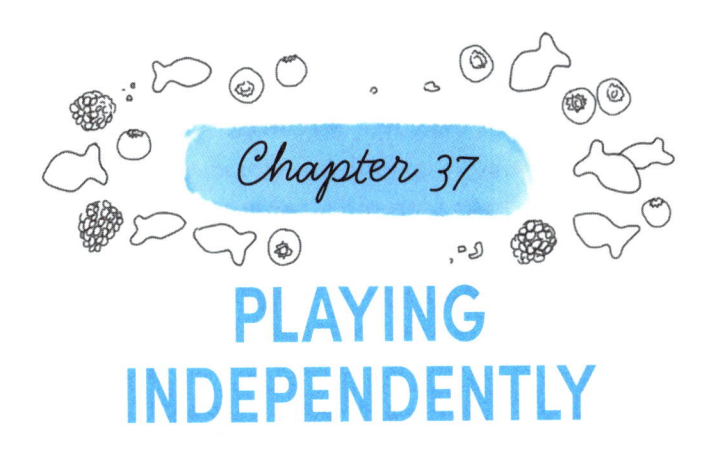

You may have heard the phrase "Play is the work of children," but it's not just a catchy saying—it's a profound truth about how toddlers learn, grow, and process the world. For toddlers, play isn't just about fun; it's the way they learn. They use play to explore their surroundings, develop social skills, solve problems, and exercise their imagination. And while *all* play is valuable, independent play is especially important. Giving your toddler the space to have unstructured play on their own fosters creativity, problem-solving, and resilience, laying the foundation for a lifetime of curiosity and confidence.

Setting the Stage for Independent Play

Kids today often face overscheduled lives, packed with school/daycare, extracurricular activities, and structured play, leaving little room for the vital kind of independent exploration that supports their well-being: **unstructured play**. Unstructured play is free, self-directed play without rigid guidelines, schedules, or adult-imposed rules. It allows children to follow their curiosity, take risks, solve problems, and develop creativity. Recent research has highlighted how the decline in unstructured playtime is closely linked to an increase in mental health challenges among children.[1] This is why independent, unstructured play is critical for healthy brain development.

When toddlers are free to explore on their own, they build critical cognitive, language, and social skills that are essential for their development. A lack of these opportunities can stifle their ability to think independently and solve problems on their own. While it comes from a place of love, the adult urge to micromanage play and pack every moment with structured activities can backfire—stifling the very independence kids need to thrive.

So how can you foster this independence while still providing a safe environment for your child to explore? Focus on simplifying your child's schedule as well as stepping back and avoiding interrupting independent play.

By letting your child explore, create, and navigate the world at a slower pace with more unstructured time, you're giving them the ultimate gift: the chance to grow and explore at their own pace.

TODDLER TIP
Don't Interrupt Independent Play

If you want your child to spend more time playing independently, stop interrupting them when you see them playing on their own. Your child is hard at work developing their concentration skills and increasing their ability to play independently.

Developmentally Appropriate Play

Tossing toys, dumping bins, or struggling to play well with others aren't "problematic" behaviors—they're completely normal and part of your child's development. These actions are often driven by **play schemas**, natural patterns of behavior toddlers engage in as they learn and make sense of the world. Jean Piaget, a key figure in cognitive development, introduced the idea of these schemas as ways children practice problem-solving, refine motor skills, and build understanding.

Here are eight common play schemas:

1. Transporting: Moving objects from one place to another (e.g., filling and dumping bins, carrying toys around).
2. Enclosing: Creating barriers or boundaries, like building walls or fences with blocks or toys.
3. Rotating: Turning things around in circles, such as spinning wheels or twirling objects.
4. Vertical Activity: Lifting or stacking things, like stacking blocks or putting items on top of one another.
5. Exploring Trajectory: Movement through space, such as dropping objects, tossing or throwing objects, running back and forth, jumping, or watching things fall.
6. Pushing/Pulling: Moving objects by pushing or pulling them (e.g., toy cars, wagons).
7. Repetition: Doing the same activity over and over again to understand cause and effect (e.g., repeatedly filling and emptying containers).
8. Hiding/Seeking: Hiding things or finding hidden objects, which helps develop object permanence.[2]

TODDLER TIP
Responding to Toy Throwing

If your child is throwing toys, it's important to get curious about the root of the behavior, then focus on meeting their needs.

> For example, if they are experimenting and exploring while practicing the trajectory schema, look for ways to give them an opportunity to throw something that is within your boundaries. This could be providing balls to toss into a basket or giving them a designated area for throwing, allowing them to explore while staying within your rules. This way, you can satisfy their need to experiment while maintaining control over the situation. If your child is throwing because they are upset, then it's important to address the feelings and emotions at the root of their behavior and teach them a better way to communicate their frustration.
>
> These schemas and stages are part of your toddler's normal growth and development. So next time your toddler is dumping everything out, remember that it's not misbehavior; it's a step in their learning journey.

Encouraging Independent Play

Independent play isn't just a break for you—it's a gift for your child. It fosters creativity, problem-solving, and self-confidence. But the reality is that independent play doesn't happen overnight. Their desire for independence is often in conflict with their need for connection. It's a dance between pushing you away while wanting you close. So how do you build up to more independent playtime?

Where to Start if You Want to Encourage Independent Play
- **Location:** Toddlers often need to be able to play near you. Set up a play area close to where you'll be, like in your home office, the living room, or even the kitchen floor while you're prepping dinner. Being close gives them the security they need to explore on their own.

TODDLER TIP
Create a "Yes Space"

If you want to encourage independent play, creating a "yes space" is essential. A yes space is a designated area where everything is safe, and your toddler is free to explore without constant micromanagement. Imagine a world where you don't have to say, "No, don't touch that" or "Be careful!" Sounds amazing, right? That's what a yes space does—it gives them the freedom to play and explore safely, and it gives you the peace of mind to let go.

- **Environment:** Focus on creating an environment that is uncluttered and organized, so it invites your child to explore rather than overwhelming them. Display toys in an accessible way, rather than tossing everything into one large bin (unless it's a bin specifically for a category of like objects). When toys are thoughtfully arranged, it encourages curiosity and independent play. Keep items at your child's height, making them easy to reach and engage with.

TODDLER TIP
Get Outdoors

In today's world, children are spending less time in nature, and that's something we can't ignore. With the rise of technology and the decrease in unstructured play, time outdoors is on the decline. Yet research shows that spending time in nature is vital for a child's

> development as it boosts creativity, problem-solving, and emotional well-being.[3] Make time to get outside regularly—whether it's a trip to the park or a nature walk—so your toddler can explore and develop essential skills in a natural setting.

- **Simple Toys:** Choose simple, open-ended toys (without battery-operated bells and whistles) like blocks, cars, magnetic tiles, dolls, and animal figurines. These are perfect for independent play because they let your toddler manipulate, create, and imagine their own scenarios. There's no "right" way to play with these toys, giving your child the freedom to explore at their own pace. Plus, these toys aren't bound to one developmental stage, so they grow with your child, adapting to their changing interests and abilities.
- **No Screens:** Keep screens out of the play area. Screen time (if you choose to use them) should be a separate activity from independent play, as it can interrupt the creativity and problem-solving skills that toddlers develop through open-ended play. Let this space be for their imagination and exploration.

ATTENTION SPAN: THE FOUNDATION OF INDEPENDENT PLAY

One of the keys to fostering independent play or setting any expectation for your toddler is understanding their attention span. Toddlers are capable of only short bursts of focus, and that's completely developmentally appropriate! As they grow, their ability to stick with an activity will increase—but they need your support along the way. By offering them opportunities to practice, you're helping them build their attention and independence, all while respecting where they are developmentally.

Age	Typical Attention Span
1 year	2–3 minutes
2 years	4–6 minutes
3 years	6–9 minutes
4 years	8–12 minutes
5 years	12–18 minutes

Start by engaging with your child for a few minutes to help them settle into the play. After five to ten minutes or so, let them know you'll be stepping away for a few moments. Depending on their age and developmental stage, you'll get different amounts of solo playtime. Make it clear that you'll come back to check on them—and do it consistently. This builds trust that you're still there, even if you're not sitting right beside them.

The Power of Sensory Play

Sensory play is one of the best ways to engage a toddler's natural curiosity and desire to explore. It stimulates their senses (sight, sound, touch, taste, and smell) and strengthens neural connections in their brain. Find ways for your child to engage in messy play (like painting, jumping in puddles, playing in mud) within your boundaries. Messy play provides kids with a rich sensory experience that is vital for their brain development.

And remember, sensory play often garners more time and engagement, but it can come with a bit more mess. Be prepared to embrace the chaos if it means longer, uninterrupted play sessions.

The great thing about sensory play is that it's often simple and doesn't require expensive materials. A bin filled with dry rice or Cheerios (taste-safe) and a few measuring cups can keep a toddler engaged for a surprisingly long time. Water play is another go-to—whether it's filling a shallow tub with water and floating small toys or giving your toddler a sponge and a bowl to squeeze water from.

Here are a few other taste-safe ideas:

- **Oobleck:** Just cornstarch and water create a fascinating texture.
- **Cold Pasta:** Cooked and chilled pasta provides a slippery, squishy sensory experience.
- **Chickpea Foam:** The liquid from a can of chickpeas (aquafaba) combined with cream of tartar creates a fun, fluffy foam.
- **Moon Dough:** Flour and oil mixed and baked create a moldable, soft dough.
- **Frozen Objects in Water:** Freeze small toys in water overnight and give your toddler warm water with a spoon or dropper to melt the ice away.

You can easily take any of these activities up a notch by adding natural food coloring for a visually stimulating twist.

Sensory Play Tips

- **Protect Your Floor:** Lay a mat under the sensory play station to protect the floor and make cleanup easier.
- **Use a Shower or Go Outside:** If you have a large shower, do water-based sensory play there, or take it outside.
- **Be Mindful of Choking Hazards:** Always watch for small objects that could be a danger.
- **Avoid Water Beads:** These can cause serious intestinal damage if swallowed. Instead, use tapioca pearls as a safe alternative.
- **Get Outside:** Walking barefoot, digging in the dirt, playing in leaves, or using a water table are all great ways to engage your child in sensory play outdoors.
- **Clean Up Together:** After play, get your toddler involved in cleaning up using a child-size broom and sponge. It teaches responsibility while keeping the fun going.

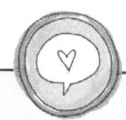

SCRIPTS FOR COMMUNICATION
Reining In Sensory Play

Scenario

Your toddler is throwing rice out of the bin.

Try

- **Stay Calm and Set a Limit:** "Rice stays in the bin." Gently guide the behavior, reinforcing the rule.
- **Follow Through:** If the behavior continues, say, "It looks like you're having trouble keeping the rice in the bin right now. We're going to take a break from the rice and try again later." Then calmly put the rice away without escalating the situation.

Remember

The break doesn't have to be long. It could be five minutes, five hours, five days, or even five months. What matters is following through. *Practice makes progress, not perfection!* Keep reinforcing the behavior you want to see, and over time, they'll learn.

TODDLER TIP
Rotate Toys

If you find your house flooded with toys, it might be time to start rotating them. Begin by removing the toys your toddler hasn't played with in the last two to three weeks. Put them away, then rotate them back in monthly or biweekly. Remember, you don't

THE PHYSICAL TODDLER

> have to rotate every single toy—two to five toys that your toddler loves or uses often can stay out. Rotating the rest will keep things fresh. A simple change in location, like moving toys from the main play area to another room, can also reinspire play and bring new excitement to familiar toys!

When *You* Don't Want to Play

Let's be honest—there are times when you just don't want to. It's okay not to want to play. You're not a bad parent if you need a break from the endless toddler games. *Play is the work of childhood, not parenthood.* While it's our job to facilitate and sometimes participate, that doesn't mean we need to be on call for playtime all day long.

It's okay to set a boundary and say, "You really want me to play with you, and I am not available right now. I'm going to do my work while you build your tower. Let me know when you've built something you want to show me!" This way, you're showing interest and support without needing to be involved in every single activity. Another option is to set a timer and say, "When the timer goes off, Mommy can play with you." Setting time limits also helps teach patience and boundaries while allowing both of you to have some space.

> ### TODDLER TIP
> *What to Do with an Early Riser*
>
> Is your little one an early riser? After your toddler goes to bed, set out a puzzle, toy, or activity that is inviting and ready to be played with first thing in the morning. This will give your child something

> exciting to engage with so you can wake up and don't have to resort to screen time first thing in the morning.

Play is serious business for toddlers. It's where they develop the skills they'll carry with them for life—creativity, problem-solving, confidence, and independence. And when you don't want to play, that's okay too. Independent play isn't just a break for you; it's a chance for your toddler to build skills and learn. Remember, you don't have to be *everything* for your child. Sometimes the best thing you can do is step back and let them take the lead, especially in play.

FAQs

Why is my toddler always dumping all their toy bins on the floor? How do I make them stop?

It could be that your child is feeling overwhelmed by their environment and can't find what they're looking for, or they may be dysregulated. Another possibility is that they're in the transporting schema, where toddlers repeatedly fill and dump bins as part of their play process. Understanding the root cause of this behavior will help you decide the best way to respond. If it's a regulation issue, helping them calm down and providing a more organized space may help. If it's part of their natural play pattern, just providing a space to engage in this behavior safely can help them learn through exploration.

How do I get my toddler to clean up their toys?

Make sure every toy has a designated spot. If there's no clear place for toys or too many are scattered around, cleanup can feel overwhelming for your child. Instead of forcing them to clean up on their own, do it with them. Modeling the process increases the likelihood that they'll join in or eventually do it on their own. Keep it fun! Turn on upbeat music or set a timer for a race to make cleaning up feel less like a chore and more like a game. You can also encourage cleaning up one toy at a time—"Let's clean up this toy before we get out another one." For younger toddlers, practice in smaller, more contained spaces like the bathtub before moving to larger areas. For older toddlers, set clear expectations, such as: "When the playroom is clean, we can go to the park. Do you want me to help you?"

How many toys should toddlers have?

On average, most toddlers do well with ten to fifteen toys out at a time. More than that can be overwhelming and actually reduce independent play. This is why toy rotation can be so helpful. Every child is different, so you'll know best what works for your little one. Keep the environment manageable and fun, and you'll see how your toddler engages with their toys in a more meaningful way.

> For a handpicked, curated list of developmentally appropriate toys by age and interest, visit transformingtoddlerhood.com/bookresources.

Part 5

THE SOCIAL TODDLER

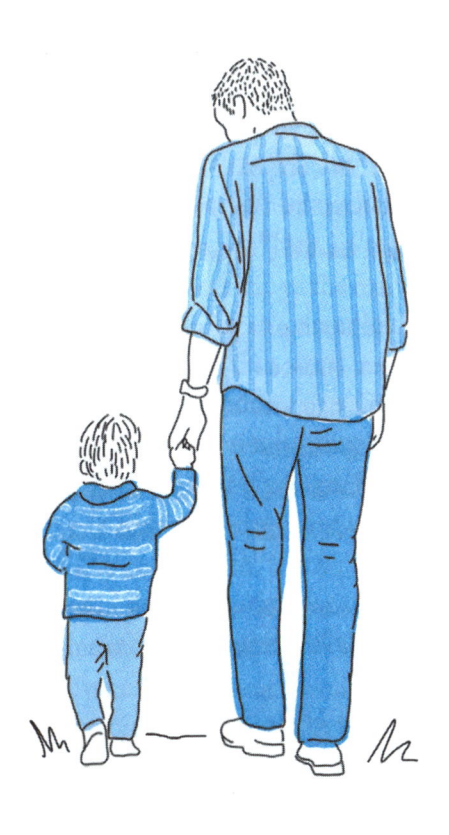

Chapter 38

MODELING MANNERS

Most parents want to raise a child who is respectful and polite, one who says "Please" and "Thank you" and willingly apologizes with an "I'm sorry" after knocking over a friend's block tower. And while it's tempting to focus on these words as markers of good behavior, real manners are about *so* much more than memorized scripts or quick apologies. They're about teaching empathy, respect, and connection while preserving your child's individuality. We want to raise children who don't just say the right words at the right time but think well, care well, and interact with confidence.

A LESSON IN MANNERS

Every moment, toddlers are absorbing how the world works by watching the people around them. We, as parents and caregivers, are their greatest teachers, and it's important not to hold kids to standards we don't hold ourselves or other adults to. And while that can feel empowering, it can also feel overwhelming. But remember: It's the little things we do every day that add up. The best way to teach your toddler manners is by modeling the

manners you want to see instead of trying to force them to do it. Here are some ideas to help you achieve that:
- Model words like *please* and *thank you* as often as you can with your child and others, and make a point to show your child how people respond to those words.
- When your child picks up their toys, help them understand this is a way of saying "thank you" to the home they live in and the people who share that space with them.
- Say "Excuse me" to your child when you need their attention. This shows them that respect goes both ways.
- Involve your child in holding doors open for others, demonstrating that helping others is a small but meaningful act of kindness.
- Smile and make eye contact with people when you interact—it's a simple but powerful way to connect.

Teaching (Not Forcing!) Apologies

We've all been there—your toddler pushes another child, grabs a toy, or says hurtful words, and before you know it, all eyes are on you, waiting for you to "do something." So you do what many parents instinctively do: You demand an apology. "Say you're sorry right now!" It's a script that most of us learned as children, but a forced apology doesn't teach what we think it does.

When we tell a child to apologize in the heat of the moment, we're teaching them to say the words but not necessarily to feel or *understand* them. In fact, forcing a child to apologize to please an adult or comply with their requests is essentially prompting a child to learn to *lie*. Your toddler may mutter a half-hearted "sorry" just to get the situation over with, but what are they learning? They're learning to appease authority, to avoid further consequences, and maybe even that *sorry* is a magic word that makes everything better, regardless of their actual feelings or the other person's experience.

This emphasis on compliance can overshadow the deeper lesson of understanding how their actions affect others. Toddlers are still developing empathy—something that typically matures around age four.[1] Expecting heartfelt apologies from a two-year-old isn't realistic. Instead, focus on teaching the meaning behind an apology by helping your child understand their actions' impact.

Forcing a child to apologize

- lacks authenticity and compassion,
- teaches that it's okay to lie about feelings,
- teaches kids to distrust their own feelings,
- doesn't address the root of the behavior,
- doesn't lead to changed behavior, and
- demands that kids pretend to be remorseful.

Instead of forcing an apology, you can try

- giving them time to calm down,
- coaching the situation,
- modeling apologizing,
- explaining what it means to apologize,
- creating teachable moments, and
- avoiding labels like "mean" and "nice."

Imagine this scenario: Your toddler is running around playing tag with a friend and pushes the other child down on the ground. The other child's parent rushes over to check on her child. She might even be glaring in your direction, expecting you to respond. First of all, don't feel pressured by other parents to respond in a certain way. Stay confident in how you choose to handle the situation and address your child thoughtfully.

Here's how a forced versus a teaching apology might play out:

Forced Apology: "That's not nice! You do not push other people. Say you're sorry right now." Sure, your toddler may go to the child and say "sorry" because he that's what he feels he needs to do to get out of trouble and continue playing. The problem is that it lacks empathy. He isn't taught to realize how his action made the other child feel.

Teaching Empathy and Modeling an Apology: Instead, you can say, "You pushed him down and now he is crying. Let's check to see if he is okay. How can you help him feel better?" This shifts the focus from compliance to compassion. You're inviting your child to understand the consequences of their actions and to take steps to make amends in a way that feels authentic. You can also model an apology: "I'm sorry you got pushed. Are you okay?" When your toddler sees you apologizing and making things right, they start to learn what an apology looks like—and more importantly, what it *feels* like. This method not only teaches empathy but helps your child develop problem-solving skills. Then you can focus on communicating the limit and what to do next time. Rather than relying on a rote apology, they're learning how to navigate complex emotions and relationships, a skill that will serve them far beyond their toddler years.

When we shift away from forcing apologies, we open the door to genuine emotional growth. Apologies are important, but only when they're rooted in real remorse. You're not just teaching them to tick a box—you're teaching them to understand the power of kindness and the importance of taking responsibility when they've hurt someone. That lesson takes time, but it's far more valuable than any forced "sorry" ever will be.

Normalize Apologizing to Your Child

It'll come as no surprise that one of the most powerful ways to teach your child about real apologies is to apologize to them when it's needed. We all have moments when we lose our cool, snap at our kids, or make a mistake. When this happens, model the same empathy and accountability you want them to learn. "I'm sorry I yelled earlier. That wasn't fair to you. Are you okay?" This simple act not only shows them what a heartfelt apology looks like, but it also reminds them that we're all learning, growing, and doing our best—just like they are.

What Happens When You Say "I'm Sorry" to a Child
- You are teaching them that you make mistakes too. No one is perfect!
- They are reminded that even adults should respect them.
- You lead by example with how to apologize.

So the next time you're tempted to demand a quick apology (or avoid an apology yourself), remember that it's not about the word; it's about the lesson. By focusing on empathy and connection, you're laying the foundation for emotional intelligence and teaching your child how to be kind, thoughtful, and aware of how their actions impact the world around them.

Handling Interruptions

If you've ever been in the middle of a conversation and your toddler starts tugging at your sleeve, chanting your name on repeat, you know the stress of toddler interruptions. It's easy to feel the urge to ignore them or snap at them to wait, but ignoring makes the behavior worse, and snapping can make your child feel bad for needing you. Toddlers live in the moment—they see, they feel, they *need*—and they haven't yet mastered the art of waiting for their turn because the part of the brain responsible for impulse control, the prefrontal cortex, is still developing. This means they lack the internal brakes to stop themselves from interrupting or demanding immediate attention when they need it or have the urge to connect. So they need us to help guide them through these moments and teach them how to wait. Here are some ideas of how to respond in the moment:

- **Connect:** "I hear you yelling 'Mommy.' You want me right now!"

- **Limit:** "I'm talking and will be done in five minutes. I'm setting the sand timer for five minutes. I can help you when it's done."
- **Follow Through** (if a child keeps interrupting): "I know it's hard to wait when you want to talk to me. The timer isn't finished yet. When it's done, I'm available."
- **Teach Skills:** "Do you want to sit on my lap or go play while you wait?" Later, in a calm moment, teach your child a better way to communicate: "When you want Mommy's attention while I'm talking, you can say 'Excuse me' or tap my hand like this. Let's practice together." Then practice—a lot. You can practice role-playing with toys and each other.
- **Keep in Mind:** Setting limits where there previously were none can trigger frustration or even meltdowns. This is normal. Your job isn't to control your child's emotions or behavior but to support them in working through their feelings while staying consistent with the limits you set. And if your child's request is something quick and manageable, consider addressing it briefly before returning to your conversation. It's okay to be flexible. This way, both needs are acknowledged, fostering a sense of cooperation and mutual respect. By practicing this approach consistently, you're teaching them to respect others' conversations without silencing their own needs or feelings. They're learning when and how to express themself.

By guiding them with these simple steps, you're helping your child build the muscle of patience. It won't happen overnight, and it certainly won't be perfect after just one reminder. But, as with anything else, practice makes progress.

In the same way, we can model patience in our own lives. When we wait calmly in a traffic jam or stand in line at the store, we're showing our children what patience looks like in real-world situations. This sets the tone when you later ask your toddler to wait their turn at the swings or during playtime. They're watching and learning from how we handle waiting, and that helps them develop this essential life skill too.

> ## TODDLER TIP
> *Help Them Understand Time*
>
> Toddlers have a poor sense of time. When we say, "In just a minute," they can struggle to understand what to expect. Help them succeed by using a visual timer. Start small—set it for one to two minutes. Say, "When the timer goes off, it's your turn." This makes time more concrete and manageable. Once they get used to short waits, gradually increase the timer length. Starting with fifteen minutes can backfire if they haven't practiced waiting—it's too abstract and might lead to frustration. Keep it simple, clear, and consistent.
>
> Over time, they'll learn the rhythm of conversations, the give and take, and the importance of waiting their turn. It's a skill they'll need for life, and it starts with you modeling patience and respect.
>
> *For a list of my favorite timers, visit transformingtoddlerhood.com/bookresources.*

Toddlers Are Learning—Not Performing

At the end of the day, teaching toddlers manners is less about external behaviors and more about building internal understanding. Your toddler doesn't need to be a mini-performer who spits out polite phrases for approval. They need to know that their feelings matter, that their voice is heard, and that kindness is about *connection*, not compliance.

So don't worry if they don't say "sorry" on command or if they interrupt you mid-sentence. Instead, focus on fostering empathy, patience, and respect, knowing your child needs a lot of practice to learn these skills. The world doesn't need more people pleasers—it needs more people who understand how to communicate with compassion and confidence. And it all starts in these early years, with you leading the way, teaching them to balance self-expression with kindness.

That's the kind of manners that matter.

FAQs

My toddler didn't want to say thank you for their birthday gifts at their party. I don't want my child to come off as ungrateful. What do I do?

If your toddler refuses to say thank you in the moment, it doesn't mean they're rude, ungrateful, or a spoiled brat. Avoid using threats like "You need to say thank you right now or you won't get more gifts!" or coercion such as "You're making Grandma sad because you didn't say thank you." These create shame and resistance.

Instead, help your child build social skills over time by practicing the following four tips:

1. **Plan Ahead:** Talk about gift giving and practice saying thank you beforehand. Role-playing is helpful.
2. **Model Gratitude:** Let your child see you expressing thanks naturally.
3. **Take Breaks:** If opening gifts becomes overwhelming, pause to help your child calm down and reconnect.
4. **Offer Alternatives:** If they can't manage words in the moment, suggest another way to show thanks, like a hug, a wave, or even a drawing later on that you put in the mail.

It's normal for toddlers to struggle with manners. They'll learn with practice.

How do I help my toddler when they forget to use their manners?

Set realistic expectations. A two-year-old might need constant reminders, while a three-year-old may remember occasionally but still need prompts. There are two ways you can be consistent about this:

1. **Practice Manners:** Use *please* and *thank you* regularly yourself.
2. **Prompt, Don't Command:** If your child says, "More toast!" respond with: "Can you ask me like this? 'More toast, please!'" Then say, "Thank you!" to recognize their effort.

Consistent modeling and positive reinforcement will help manners become a habit.

Chapter 39

ADDRESSING LYING

Your toddler's first fib might catch you off guard—but it's not a cause for alarm. In fact, it's a powerful sign that their brain is growing in remarkable ways. By around age three, your child starts realizing, "Hey, you don't know everything that's in my head!" This newfound awareness sparks a wave of experimentation, including stretching the truth or crafting imaginative tales.

Maybe they insist the wind knocked over the vase or swear their sibling broke the toy that was clearly in their hands moments before. These creative stories aren't about being bad or deceptive; they're about discovery. Your toddler is learning how minds work, and that realization is a big leap in their cognitive and emotional development. The ability to lie, surprisingly, is a cognitive milestone worth celebrating, as it marks the beginning of understanding perspective, intention, and individuality.

Why Do Toddlers Lie?

Kids don't lie because they're bad or manipulative; often they're testing boundaries and trying to figure out how the world works. They lie because they're scared, embarrassed, confused, or trying to avoid getting into trouble—and sometimes they're simply engaging in fantasy play! A toddler's imagination is wild, and the line between what's real and what's imagined is quite blurry until around the age of six.

Punishing or shaming your child for lying might stop the behavior temporarily—but at the cost of long-term trust. How you handle lying in toddlerhood shapes whether your child will trust you when life gets complicated down the road. If you want a teenager who comes to you when they've messed up or when they're in a risky situation, you need to show your toddler now that honesty is always safer than hiding the truth. This means not punishing your child for lying.

Labeling kids as "liars" or punishing them can backfire, leading to even more lying, not less. Why? Because fear of punishment triggers survival instincts, making a child more likely to lie to escape perceived danger. Creating a safe space where honesty is met with understanding, not shame, builds trust and strengthens your connection—now and in the future.

Responding to Lying

When you catch your toddler in a lie, resist the urge to scold and punish. Instead, get curious. Ask yourself, *What is this lie trying to protect?* Maybe they were afraid you'd be mad. Maybe they didn't realize it was safe to tell the truth. Your job isn't just to correct the lie—it's to help them feel secure enough to be honest, even when the truth is hard.

Focus on setting clear limits while staying calm and supportive. Partner with your child to figure out what happened, why they lied, and how they can handle it differently next time. This approach keeps the focus on problem-solving, not punishment, strengthening trust and connection.

SCRIPTS FOR COMMUNICATION
Responding to Lying

Avoid Saying: "Lying is bad. Don't lie to me."
Try Saying: "I know that's not what happened. It's okay to tell me the truth—you won't be in trouble. Let's figure this out together."

> This approach reassures your child that honesty is safe, even when they've made a mistake.

By responding with curiosity and compassion, you create a space where your child learns that your love and support aren't conditional on getting everything right.

The Recipe for More Honesty

So how do you encourage honesty? It starts with safety and trust.

Create a Safe Environment for Truth

When your toddler tells the truth, make sure they know it's okay—even if they've done something they shouldn't have. Instead of reacting with frustration, acknowledge their honesty and focus on what comes next. For example, you might say, "Thank you for telling me the truth that you spilled the juice. Let's clean it up together."

This shows your child that being honest doesn't lead to punishment but rather partnership. You're solving problems with them, not against them.

Don't Prompt a Lie

If you know your child did something, don't set them up to lie by asking a yes/no question: "Did you get water all over the bathroom floor?" Instead, say something like: "There is water all over the bathroom floor. Water stays in the sink. Let's go clean it up together."

Validate Their Emotions

Toddlers often lie when they feel overwhelmed or afraid. Instead of focusing on the lie, acknowledge what might be going on beneath the surface. Say something like: "I wonder if you were worried I'd be upset about the marker on the wall. I know it was an accident, and we can fix it together. Next time, marker stays on the paper."

By addressing the emotions behind the behavior, you show your child that honesty is emotionally safe.

Teach Accountability Without Fear

Kids need to learn that their actions have consequences, but they don't need to learn it through fear. When a child tells a lie, guide them through taking responsibility in a supportive way. For instance: "I know the toy broke when you were playing with it. It's okay to tell me the truth. What can you do differently next time so this doesn't happen again?" This helps them learn responsibility in a way that doesn't feel punishing but rather empowering.

Model Honesty Yourself

Children mimic what they see, and they're always watching how you respond to situations. Be mindful of your own honesty, even in little moments. If they catch you telling a small fib (like telling someone you're "busy" when you're not), take the time to explain. "You heard me tell Daddy I'm too busy to play, but really, I just need a break. It's important to be honest, so I'll tell him the truth." This shows your toddler that honesty is a value you hold dear—and one they'll want to emulate.

The Long Game

Encouraging honesty in your toddler is a long game. It's about building a relationship based on trust, respect, and open communication. By creating an environment where your child feels safe to be truthful, you're laying the groundwork for lifelong honesty. Parenting is a marathon, not a sprint.

Remember, lying at this age is not a character flaw—it indicates a developmental milestone. Our response to it is what shapes their future understanding of honesty. So when your child experiments with bending the truth, take a deep breath, lean into connection, and show them that honesty is always worth it.

FAQs

What should I say when my child denies something obvious, even when the evidence is right there?

Toddlers often deny wrongdoing when they fear getting in trouble or feel overwhelmed by guilt or embarrassment. By calmly acknowledging what you see and inviting them to solve the problem together, you shift the focus from blame to collaboration. This reduces defensiveness and encourages them to take responsibility. You're showing that mistakes are part of learning, not something to fear or hide. Try this: "I hear you saying you didn't touch the lamp. I can see that it's on the floor now. It's okay to tell me what happened so we can fix it together." Focus on solving the problem, not assigning blame. This approach encourages honesty without making them feel cornered.

How do I respond when my child tells an outlandish story that clearly isn't true?

Toddlers live in a world where reality and imagination often blend. Their stories might seem like lies, but they're often a creative way of processing experiences. By acknowledging the imaginative tale, you validate their creativity while gently steering them toward honesty. This keeps the conversation light, avoids shame, and models how to separate fact from fiction respectfully. Say something like: "Wow! That's an interesting story. Sometimes our imaginations can run wild. Please tell me what really happened so we can figure it out." This response guides them back to reality with curiosity, not criticism.

Chapter 40

EASING SEPARATION ANXIETY

Your toddler's world revolves around you, and they depend on you to meet not only their physical needs but also their emotional ones. This can make it incredibly challenging for your toddler to part from you—whether it's at bedtime, daycare, when you leave for work, or during a night out. For them, separation can feel like the end of the world—a sudden, deep ache that tugs at their tiny hearts and sets off waves of distress. While separation anxiety is a common part of toddlerhood, the good news is that it's temporary, manageable, and—believe it or not—something you can help your child navigate with greater ease.

What Is Separation Anxiety?

Separation anxiety is when a child becomes agitated and upset when a parent tries to leave, often resulting in tears, protests, and tantrums. It typically appears several times during infancy and toddlerhood. It can ebb and flow as they grow, intensifying at times due to changes like starting daycare, developmental shifts, or even feeling tired or unwell. For some kids, their personality and temperament make them more prone to separation anxiety. While it's a completely normal part of development, it doesn't make it any easier when your toddler clings to your leg like you're their lifeline at drop-off time. This doesn't mean something is wrong—it's a sign of secure attachment, a reflection of the love and security you've worked so hard to build.

> ### TODDLER TIP
> *Practice Separation*
>
> Help ease your toddler's separation anxiety by practicing short, positive separations ahead of time. Start with brief separations while leaving your toddler with a trusted, loving adult, gradually increasing the time apart as they adjust. "Daddy is going to leave for a little while, and Grandma will stay with you. I'll be back after snack time." These practice runs build trust and reinforce the important lesson that *you will always come back*. With each successful reunion, your toddler's confidence grows, helping them feel more secure when the real goodbyes happen.
>
> *What to Avoid*
> - **Dismissing and Fixing Feelings:** "Don't cry. You're fine. You're going to have so much fun at school/with Grandma!"
>
> *What to Try Instead*
> - **Validation and Reassurance:** "You want Daddy to stay. I know. It's hard to leave Daddy. I will be back after naptime!"

Supporting Your Child in Separating

So how do you help your toddler when they feel like your departure is the end of their world? Here's a step-by-step guide to managing separation anxiety, especially during daycare or preschool drop-offs:

1. **Prepare in Advance:** Talk to your toddler about what's going to happen. Even at a young age, children benefit from hearing what the day will look like: "We're going to daycare, and after you play with your friends and have snack time, Mommy will be back to pick you up."
2. **Create a Goodbye Routine:** Rituals can be a lifesaver. Whether it's a special hug, a high five, or a silly handshake, having a consistent way of saying goodbye helps your child feel more secure. It signals that while you're leaving, everything is okay.
3. **Be Calm and Confident:** Kids pick up on your energy. If you're anxious or hesitant about leaving, they'll sense it. Model confidence and let them know that this is a regular part of life. Offer your love and reassurance, but don't linger too long—it can make the goodbye harder.
4. **Acknowledge Their Feelings:** It's okay to validate their emotions: "I know it's hard to say goodbye, and you're feeling sad." Teaching them to express their feelings without being dismissed helps them build emotional resilience.
5. **Be Specific:** Saying "I'll be home later" or "I'll be back by four" doesn't mean much to a child because it's not very concrete and toddlers can't tell time. So put it in terms that your child can understand: "I'll be back before lunch!"
6. **Stay Consistent:** Even when drop-offs feel like they're spiraling into a pattern of tears, consistency is key. Stick to your routine and remind your child of the return time. The predictability helps soothe their anxiety.
7. **Use a Comfort Object:** Encourage your toddler to take something familiar from home, like a stuffed animal or blanket, to daycare. This small comfort can act as a bridge between home and the new environment. You can also offer something personal from yourself, like a scarf or bracelet, to help them feel connected. Another idea is to put matching heart stamps on both your hand and theirs, creating a visible reminder of your bond. Consider placing a family photo in your child's bag for them to look at whenever they need a sense of reassurance.

8. **Say Goodbye:** As tempting as it may be to sneak out while they're playing, don't. Sneaking away might avoid the meltdown in the moment, but when your child finally realizes you've gone, their trust gets shaken. They may start to feel unsure about when you might disappear again, leading to even more intense separation anxiety the next time. Even if it leads to tears, it's essential to create a predictable routine that teaches your toddler that you'll always come back.

9. **Reassess the Environment:** Sometimes the intensity of the separation anxiety is a sign that the environment might not be the best fit for your child. If your toddler's distress seems overwhelming and doesn't ease over time, it could be worth considering whether the setting is nurturing enough for their needs. Are the caregivers nurturing? Is the environment too loud? Too bright? Look for ways to accommodate your child's needs.

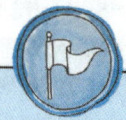

RED FLAG
When to Talk to a Doctor

Separation anxiety is expected during toddlerhood, but if your child's anxiety feels extreme—causing physical symptoms like stomachaches, nightmares, or significant behavioral changes—it's worth speaking to a pediatrician or child psychologist. They can help determine whether this is a normal developmental phase or if additional support is needed.

Transitioning Your Toddler to Daycare or Preschool

Transitioning to daycare or preschool is one of the most common triggers for separation anxiety. It's helpful to prepare in advance. The older the child is, the longer runway you should create for the transition—about five to seven days for a one-to-two-year-old and two weeks for a three- or four-year-old. However, you know your child best!

Tips for Transitioning

- **Visit the School Together:** Before the first official drop-off, bring your toddler to visit the daycare or preschool. Let them explore the space, meet the teachers, and get a feel for the environment with you there as a safety net.
- **Practice:** Give your child gradual exposure by driving past the school or practicing the new morning routine together. Role-play drop-off scenarios to help your toddler know what to expect. This makes the process feel more familiar and less intimidating.
- **Read Books:** Reading books about daycare or preschool can open up conversations about what's coming. Use books as tools to spark curiosity, address concerns, and normalize the experience. The more familiar the concept, the less daunting it will seem.
- **Give a Sense of Control:** Let your child choose their backpack, lunchbox, or even a small comfort item to bring. Allowing age-appropriate choices gives them a sense of control within set boundaries, which helps reduce feelings of powerlessness.
- **Transfer to a Trusted Adult:** When dropping off, always hand your child directly to a familiar teacher or caregiver. Use reassuring language: "Here is Miss Smith. She's going to take care of you today." This creates a bridge of trust, making the transition less overwhelming than leaving them alone in a busy classroom.
- **Start with Short Stays:** If the daycare allows, begin with shorter stays and gradually increase the time your child spends there. This approach builds trust and comfort with the new routine, helping your child adjust at their own pace.
- **Talk About It Daily:** Make daycare or preschool a normal topic of conversation. Ask open-ended questions about what your child thinks or feels. Encouraging them to express their inner thoughts helps you address concerns and ease fears through supportive conversations.

- **Give It Time:** Adjustment takes time. Some kids bounce back within a week, others need more time to settle. Patience is key.

Even though separation anxiety may feel overwhelming, it's a typical part of development. With developmentally appropriate tools and plenty of empathy, you can help your toddler transition through this phase with more confidence and ease. And when the time comes, those tearful drop-offs will be replaced by excited waves and laughter. In the end, this, too, shall pass, and with it, your child will grow stronger, more independent, and more secure in the knowledge that you'll always come back.

FAQs

How long does separation anxiety last?

Separation anxiety varies from child to child. Some experience several bouts, while for others, it's a brief phase. It typically peaks between 18 months and 2.5 years. The good news is that for most children, separation anxiety fades by age 3 or 4 as they develop a stronger sense of independence. However, it can resurface during big transitions, like starting daycare or preschool, moving to a new home, or adjusting to a new sibling. Every child is unique, so timelines can differ.

Why is my toddler so clingy all of a sudden?

Toddlers can go through clingy stages where they seem to need you every second—wanting to be held constantly and getting upset if you step away even for a moment. This is often triggered by developmental leaps, illness, fatigue, or major changes in their environment. The more we try to push them away during these stages, the more it can heighten their separation fears, making them cling even tighter. Instead, approach these moments with empathy while setting gentle boundaries: "Mommy needs to go to the bathroom. I'm going to put you down, and I'll pick you up when I'm done." If your child cries, acknowledge their feelings while holding firm: "I hear you crying. You really want Mommy to hold you. I'm almost done, and I'll be right back to pick you up." Separation doesn't have to be tear-free to be supportive and respectful. Each time you follow through, you're showing them that even when you go, *you always come back*.

How do I talk to my toddler about the death of a family member, especially if it triggers separation anxiety?

Use simple, honest, age-appropriate language: "Grandpa died, which means his body stopped working, and we won't see him anymore." Avoid confusing and vague terms like *gone to sleep* or *passed away*. Validate their feelings: "I know you're sad. I miss Grandpa too." Ask, "What questions do you have?" Reassure them they are safe and loved, and answer their questions patiently, even if they repeat them.

How can I support my toddler's separation anxiety during a divorce, deployment, and other separations?

Be clear and consistent: "Mommy and Daddy live in different houses, but we both love you, and you'll see us both." Stick to routines to provide comfort and predictability. Validate their feelings: "I know this is not what you wanted. I'm here to help you." Reassure them often that they are safe and loved. Create a visual countdown until they will see the other parent, using sticky notes on the wall or drawing boxes to check off on a piece of paper. Consider recording a voice note of that parent reading a favorite book that you can play during reading time. Utilize video chat (if possible) or hang a photo of the parent at your child's level.

Chapter 41

SUPPORTING A SLOW-TO-WARM-UP (SHY) CHILD

It's your toddler's birthday party, and the house is buzzing with excitement. Guests are arriving, presents in hand, and Aunt Sara cheerfully says, "Say hello!" to the birthday star. Their eyes drop, their little hand tightens around yours, and you can feel the tension radiating off them as they desperately cling to your leg. What do you do? The social pressure is on. All eyes are on you to "fix" the situation. But forcing your child to say hello will not make them more likely to do so next time. In fact, it might just backfire and create a power struggle that leaves you both feeling frustrated and misunderstood.

Raise your hand if you've been there. And keep it raised if you've ever felt the sting of embarrassment when your toddler refuses to engage in a simple greeting, leaving you fumbling for words or feeling like maybe you've dropped the ball on teaching manners. But let me tell you this—there's absolutely nothing wrong with your child or your parenting.

The reality is that every child comes into this world with their own unique lens for how they approach new experiences, and this lens is called their *temperament*. Some kids waltz into new situations without a second thought, while others hang back, observing quietly from the sidelines.

Neither approach is better or worse; it's simply the way they're wired. And when you have a child who is slow to warm up, it's important to see their hesitance not as a flaw but as a natural part of who they are.

Don't Label—Empower

One of the most crucial things you can do as a parent is to avoid labeling your child as "shy." Labels stick. Even though "shy" might seem harmless, it can quickly become a limiting identity. Every time you or someone else says, "Oh, she's just shy," your child hears it, absorbs it, and may begin to see themselves that way. It reinforces the very behavior you're hoping to change.

In fact, according to the University of Nevada, "When children are given labels, it affects not only the way they see themselves but also what is expected of them and how they are treated, which in turn, influences who they become." Labels—even positive ones—can affect children's sense of self and limit their potential.[1]

When a toddler won't say hello to a friend, family member, or stranger on command, it does *not* mean they are rude or disrespectful. It means they are feeling unsure and aren't comfortable enough yet. Labeling a child as rude or disrespectful comes from seeing behavior through a binary lens of good/bad or right/wrong, which oversimplifies what's really happening and fails to consider that behavior is communication.

Helping your toddler feel comfortable with a visitor happens when they are allowed to stay with and be supported by their safe and secure base in the beginning, until connection is created with the new person. Once connection is established, your toddler will feel more comfortable interacting with that person, including talking to them.

What's important is to *honor where your child is at*. Respecting their feelings and fears looks like saying, "It's okay to take your time. You can stay with me until you're ready to play." Creating a sense of connection and security will encourage your child to explore with confidence, knowing you're there when they need you.

> ### TODDLER TIP
> *Identify Feelings*
>
> When your child seems slow to warm up, there's a big difference between saying, "You're shy!" and "I wonder if you're feeling shy." The first statement labels your child, which can stick and shape how they see themself. The second helps them identify and understand their emotions, fostering self-awareness without assigning a fixed identity. This small shift builds emotional intelligence while leaving room for growth and change!

Tools for Supporting a Slow-to-Warm-Up Child

Now let's get practical. How can you support your child in navigating new situations without reinforcing their hesitance or labeling them as shy? Here are some actionable steps:

Step 1: Prepare Them Ahead of Time

Children who are slow to warm up thrive on predictability. Before heading into a new situation, talk to your child about what to expect. For example: "We're going to Aunt Sara's house, and there will be a lot of people there." Mention who will be there specifically and what everyone will be doing. Ask your toddler what they want to do while they're there and help them come up with a simple plan.

Arrive early if possible. Being one of the first people there can feel much less intimidating than walking into a room full of people when the event is already in full swing. This approach helps your child feel prepared, supported, and empowered to engage at their own pace.

Step 2: Role-Play Social Situations

Practice makes progress, right? Use stuffed animals or dolls to act out different social scenarios with your child. Give them the opportunity to rehearse saying hello, making eye contact, or asking to join a game. This builds their confidence in a safe and playful setting.

Step 3: Offer Them Choices

Instead of forcing your child to say hello or engage in a particular way, offer them choices. Ask, "Would you like to wave or give a high five?" or "Would you like to play with the kids now or sit with me and watch for a little while?" Giving your child choices lets them feel a sense of control in the situation, reducing the pressure to perform on command. You can also gently guide them into participation by getting involved yourself. For example, at a party, you might say, "There are lots of fun things to do! Should we get our faces painted or grab something to eat first?" This approach makes engaging feel less like a requirement and more like a shared adventure.

Step 4: Celebrate the Small Wins

When your child does take a small step—whether it's making eye contact, waving, or simply standing closer to the group—acknowledge it. You might say, "I noticed you watched the kids for a while, then you decided to join in. You did it!" This helps your child recognize their own progress without feeling overwhelmed by expectations.

Step 5: Look for Opportunities to Practice

Provide opportunities for your child to practice social interactions in low-pressure settings. Start with activities your child already enjoys, then gently invite another child to join in. Consider structured activities like a parent/caregiver music class, where social interaction is guided but not forced. These settings allow your child to observe, engage at their own pace, and gradually build social confidence in a supportive environment.

SCRIPTS FOR COMMUNICATION
Warming Up "Shy" Children

Forcing a child to say hello sends the message, "Saying hello right now is more important than your feelings, emotions, and needs." Instead, small shifts in language can create space for your child to grow and adapt without feeling boxed into a role they're not ready to play.

Avoid Saying	*Try Saying*
"I'm sorry she won't say hi."	"She's not ready to say hello yet." Or "She will come say hello when she is ready."
"She's shy."	"She is still deciding whether she is comfortable."
"You need to say hello."	"You really want her to say hello, and she's not ready."
"I don't know why she does this. Her sister is so social."	"She's observing right now and that's okay."
"Stop being rude and say hi."	"How do you want to say hello? Would you like to wave or high-five to say hello?"
"You need to say hello to Grandma. She came here to play with you."	"Grandma is excited to see you. Let's go show her your blocks."

These gentle language shifts show respect for your child's boundaries while encouraging social engagement on their terms.

Trust the Process

Remember, every child moves at their own pace. Some kids are naturally more reserved, and that's perfectly okay. What matters most is that your child feels supported and understood. By honoring their temperament, creating a sense of safety, and offering gentle encouragement, you'll help your slow-to-warm-up child find their confidence in their own time.

So the next time your child clings to your leg at a family gathering or sits on the bench watching other kids play, take a deep breath and remind yourself: *This isn't a race.* With patience, understanding, and connection, your child will eventually step into the world on their terms. And when they do, you'll be right there, cheering them on.

FAQs

How do I respond when family members and friends call my child shy?

As a parent, it's your job to remind your family and friends that your toddler gets to decide when and how they interact and show affection. It's your job to do what's best for your child and to give them the tools they need to navigate social situations. You might respond, "She's unsure and deciding if she feels comfortable." You can set the record straight in a way that respects everyone.

What if my child never warms up at a gathering or says hello or goodbye?

It's okay if your child doesn't warm up at a social event. Respect their comfort level and avoid pressuring them. Consistently model social behavior without forcing it. Say, "I'm going to say hello now" or "We're leaving—let's say goodbye!" This shows your child what's expected while letting them learn through observation. Social confidence builds over time with patience and support.

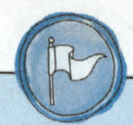

RED FLAG
Social and Communication Challenges

If your child consistently avoids interaction, shows extreme distress in social settings, or struggles to communicate their needs, consider speaking with a pediatrician or child development specialist for guidance.

Chapter 42

MANAGING SIBLING CONFLICT

Sibling conflict—it's unavoidable. You've seen it all: whining and shouts of "That's not fair!" plus pushing, hitting, and endless accusations. In those moments, your instinct is to step in, take control, and referee the chaos. Restore the peace. End the fight.

But your greatest power as a parent isn't in playing referee; it's in being the coach. A referee enforces rules and calls out infractions, but a coach teaches the players how to solve problems, strategize, and work together.

When it comes to sibling conflict, that's where your strength lies—empowering your kids with the skills they need to resolve their own disputes. These aren't just survival tactics for childhood—they're essential relationship and conflict-resolution skills that will serve them well long after the shouting has faded. Here's a step-by-step guide to managing sibling conflict.

Step 1: Establish Safety

When sibling conflict escalates into physical aggression—pushing, hitting, grabbing—it's critical to step in and ensure everyone's physical safety. This doesn't mean jumping into referee mode, issuing punishments, or deciding who's right or wrong. It simply means creating a safe environment where each child can begin to regulate their emotions and, in turn, their behavior.

If necessary, physically separate the kids—especially if they are having trouble controlling their bodies or are too upset to calm down together. This might mean standing between them or gently guiding one to another space, like the couch or a nearby room. The goal isn't isolation but creating a safe space where they can start to regulate their emotions

Once *physical safety* is ensured, it's crucial to focus on *emotional safety*. Start with yourself—take a deep breath and get centered before you help your children regulate their emotions. Your calm presence will guide them toward calmness. Remember, check on both children, not just the one who is crying. Both kids are affected by the situation and need your physical and emotional support. Sit down and put your arm around each child, offering comfort to both. This lets them know you're there for them and that their feelings matter.

Say something like, "I can see you're really upset. I'm here." This helps both children feel supported and understood. Your soothing words and actions help create a safe emotional space where they can begin to process their feelings and prepare for the next steps in resolving the conflict.

Step 2: Build Connection and Set Limits

Start by getting curious and opening the dialogue with a neutral description of what happened: "I walked in and you were standing there with your toy and crying. What happened?" This simple question invites your child to share their perspective, showing them you're interested in understanding their feelings. Give each child an opportunity to share (if they can) and be sure to validate their experience. Validation does not mean you are condoning a behavior. Instead you are soothing emotions by creating connection.

Once everyone feels seen and heard, it's time to set the limit. Use a calm, firm voice: "It's okay to want your own space. *And* hitting hurts. It's unsafe." By setting a clear limit, you let your child know that while their feelings are valid, certain behaviors are not acceptable. This combination of connection and limits gives your child the security of feeling understood while also reinforcing the importance of respect and appropriate actions.

Step 3: Use Coaching Conflict-Resolution Skills

This is where you guide your children in learning conflict-resolution skills. But here's an important reminder: We teach these skills when kids are calm, not at the height of the upset. When emotions are running high, it's not the right time to try to solve the problem or teach a lesson. Instead, focus on helping them calm down first. Once they've settled, that's when you can guide them through problem-solving and teach them the tools they need to resolve conflicts on their own. The goal is to empower them with the skills to handle disagreements independently, without always needing you to step in and fix things. Of course, this won't happen right away, but with repetition and practice, you'll be surprised at how much progress they make.

TODDLER TIP
Be a Coach

Instead of being the judge and jury during sibling conflict, practice being the coach to support your kids in building their relationship. If we come in as the judge and jury, kids don't learn the skills they need to navigate conflict, and the responsibility to solve their problems always falls on you. The goal is to work yourself out of the job as you transfer the skills to your children and build them.

Developing Conflict-Resolution Skills

Let's break down a few essential skills that can support your children into becoming problem-solvers. Remember, teaching and practicing new skills should happen in the calm moments.

Impulse Control

One of the biggest challenges kids face during conflict is controlling their impulses—especially when emotions are running high. You've likely seen this in the form of hitting, grabbing, or pushing. The goal here is to help your child slow down and find more appropriate ways to communicate.

Script: "Next time you are feeling frustrated and want to hit, what can you do instead? Let's practice." Note: You might have to give younger toddlers ideas of what they can do instead. Older toddlers will likely have plenty of ideas of their own!

The goal here is to help them recognize that while their feelings are valid, their actions need to be safe.

Script: "That's so frustrating, *and* hitting hurts. It's unsafe. What can you do instead when you're upset?"

Over time, your child will learn to pause before reacting, giving them space to make a better choice in the future.

Effective Communication

Often, sibling conflict escalates because kids don't have the words to express how they feel, so they lash out physically or verbally. Teaching them to articulate their emotions is crucial.

Script: "How did you feel when she grabbed your toy? Let's tell her. Say, 'I feel upset when you grab my toys.'"

It's also important to teach kids how to communicate using signs or gestures. This can be especially effective for younger toddlers who might not have fully developed verbal skills.

Script: "When you want your brother to stop, put your hand up like this and say, 'Stop, please.'"

By introducing these communication tools, you help children express their needs in a clear, nonconfrontational way. Encouraging communication between siblings not only helps them articulate their feelings but also ensures they feel heard. This skill reduces frustration and leads to quicker, more peaceful resolutions—teaching your children the power of words over actions in handling conflict.

Joint Solutions

Conflict resolution is about more than just stating your feelings—it's about finding solutions that work for everyone involved. Teach older toddlers how to brainstorm ideas and reach compromises. Encourage them to think creatively and come up with win-win solutions. For example, "What can we do so both of you can enjoy playing here?" or "I wonder what we can do to solve this. How can you work this out together?" This allows them to practice problem-solving skills and take ownership of their disagreements. If you have a younger toddler and a baby, you can still guide them through this process with your own ideas, as they won't be able to answer.

Calm and Regulation

In the middle of a conflict, staying calm is critical, and it's a skill children can learn with practice. In a calm moment, teach them skills to help manage their emotions in the heat of the moment.

Script: "When I feel upset, it helps me to take deep breaths and count to three. Let's practice together. How does that make you feel?"

This simple exercise can help your child calm down enough to move past their big emotions and focus on finding a solution. And over time, they'll learn how to regulate themself in moments of stress.

TODDLER TIP
Increasing the Sibling Bond

Avoid comparing siblings to each other, pitting them against each other, or talking negatively about one sibling in front of another. This can break down the sibling relationship and fuel sibling rivalry.

Setting the Stage for Lifelong Problem-Solvers

Conflict resolution is a skill that takes time to build. The younger a child is, the more support they'll need. It's essential to remember that kids who are in the middle of emotional upset aren't ready to move forward and find solutions right away.

Your first job is to separate them enough to create safety and support them as they move through their big emotions. Only then can they begin learning how to resolve the conflict. And this learning process takes time, repetition, and practice. If it feels like it's not working, you might ask yourself, *What skills does my child need to learn to be successful here?* or *What support does my child need to follow through?*

Focus on one thing at a time. Maybe it's practicing impulse control today or helping them communicate better tomorrow. With each conflict, you're giving them the tools they need to solve problems themselves. Eventually, you'll see them use those tools without needing you to step in at all.

So the next time you see a toy flying through the air or witness a disagreement escalating, take a deep breath and remember: You're not the referee in this game. You're the coach, and your kids are learning to play with confidence and kindness, one conflict at a time.

FAQs

My child keeps saying "That's not fair!" What do I do?

When your child says, "That's not fair," listen to their feelings and validate them. "You feel like that's not fair." Be patient and stay with them until they start to calm down. Once they're more settled, explain that "fair" doesn't always mean the same or equal—it means meeting everyone's needs. Get curious about the emotions and needs beneath their words. What are they really feeling? Are they feeling overlooked or frustrated? Focus on soothing those emotions and meeting those needs, all while staying within your boundaries.

My toddlers are always fighting, and I feel like I've tried everything. What can I do?

First, take a moment to reflect on how you're responding. Are you accidentally reinforcing the fighting by picking sides or labeling one child as "the problem" and the other as "the victim"? These labels can fuel challenging behavior. Next, consistently apply coaching techniques, like those mentioned above, to help them navigate their disagreements. Give it at least two weeks before reassessing the situation.

Get curious about what's driving the behavior. Is one child feeling jealous? Is one struggling with impulse control? Don't be afraid to separate them if needed. You can say, "Looks like you're having trouble playing together right now. It's best if you take a break from each other. We'll try playing again later." Then, guide them to find separate activities in different areas. During the calm moments, work on strengthening the sibling bond through shared positive experiences. Keep focusing on building that connection and reinforcing the skills they need to resolve conflicts.

Chapter 43

CULTIVATING SHARING SKILLS

Every parent knows the playtime battlefield: toys scattered, kids happily playing—until that one fateful moment when your child notices a friend holding *their* toy. Suddenly, it's a showdown of possession, and you're stuck in the middle, trying to referee.

Here's the thing: Toddlers see the world through a *me-centered* lens. Developmentally, they're wired to believe that everything in their environment is connected to them. So when they spot a sibling or friend playing with something from *their* toy bin, their brain immediately sounds the alarm: *Wait a second—that's my toy! Why are they playing with it? I want it now!*

While this reaction can be frustrating, it's developmentally appropriate. A child's ability to share isn't about being "nice" or "mean"—it's about where they are developmentally. Children under three cannot grasp the concept of sharing.[1] In fact, experts explain that real sharing skills typically don't appear until closer to age four, when the brain's prefrontal cortex starts to mature more rapidly.[2]

Why? Because toddlers are still figuring out big stuff like impulse control, empathy, and even realizing that other people have feelings too. To them, "me, mine, now" isn't selfish—it's instinctual! Expecting a young child to share is like expecting them to read before they know the sounds letters make—it's simply not a skill they've developed yet. Understanding this can help you drop unrealistic expectations and focus on coaching them toward sharing when their brains are ready.

There's a massive difference between *making* kids share and *teaching* them to share. And when it comes down to it, forced sharing causes more challenges than it is helpful.

Forced Sharing vs. Child-Led Turn-Taking

It's easy to fall into the trap of forcing a child to share—especially when you're trying to avoid a meltdown from the child left wanting. **Forced sharing** happens when adults step in to manage the giving and taking of toys, dictating when and how children must share. It's an externally driven, adult-controlled process—often referred to as "sharing on demand."

Imagine your child is happily playing with a doll when another child comes over and demands a turn. You step in and say, "You've had it long enough. It's their turn now." Or you set a timer, and when it goes off, you make your child hand over the toy, whether they're ready or not.

Why Forced Sharing Backfires

While this might seem like a quick fix to avoid conflict or a way to teach kindness, it comes with unintended consequences that can hinder your child's social and emotional development and do more harm than good. Forced sharing backfires for the following different reasons:

For the Child Who Wants the Toy
- It rewards behavior that is not pro-social.
- It encourages instant gratification.
- It creates a missed opportunity to practice impulse control.
- It teaches the child to rely on adults to solve their problems.

For the Child Who Is Playing with the Toy
- It teaches that what they are doing isn't important.
- It takes away their voice and ability to stand up for themself.
- It encourages people-pleasing.
- It communicates that the needs and feelings of others are more important than their own.

When sharing is forced, toddlers don't actually learn the deep-rooted social skills we want them to master. Instead, they learn compliance. Sure, the other kid gets the truck, but at what cost? Your child may feel resentful, confused, and powerless. And resentment doesn't foster compassion—it fosters resistance.

Imagine you're scrolling on your phone, fully engrossed—maybe reading an article, answering a text, or watching a video—and suddenly, your boss or partner walks up and says, "Okay, that's enough. Now hand your phone over to so-and-so. It's their turn." How would you feel? Frustrated? Annoyed? A little disrespected?

That's exactly how your child feels when they're told to give up a toy they're not done with. To them, that toy is their *important work*—their connection, their focus, their joy in the moment. When we interrupt that and force sharing, we're not just taking away a toy; we're undermining their sense of autonomy and respect.

So what's the alternative to forcing a child to share? **Child-led turn-taking.**

The Benefits of Child-Led Turn-Taking

Child-led turn-taking allows children to decide when they're finished playing with a toy before passing it along. It's their turn until they're done. If a toy is being played with, it's simply *not* available for someone else yet. If no one is playing with it, then it's available. This is a concrete explanation that young children can understand. It's driven by an *internal* sense of readiness rather than *external* adult control. This approach respects both the child playing and the one waiting by teaching impulse control, conflict-resolution skills, and intrinsic generosity over people-pleasing.

Let's take that same example and imagine your child is playing with a doll when another child walks up, eager for a turn. Instead of stepping in and demanding your child share, you say, "She's playing with the doll right now. It's not available. You can have a turn when she's done."

By waiting, the second child learns that patience pays off and that others' playtime matters too. When the first child eventually finishes and willingly hands over the doll, they experience the joy of sharing on *their* terms—not because an adult forced them to.

It might seem subtle, but this shift from compliance-based, forced sharing to turn-taking led by the child is game-changing. Instead of swooping in as the referee of the toy squabble, you become a guide, helping your toddler understand the flow of play, the idea of waiting, and, most importantly, the joy of generosity that comes from within, not from being told what to do. Also, often children will easily give up the toy once they no longer feel the threat of losing it. Unlike forced sharing, which is about maintaining adult-imposed peace, child-led turn-taking is about teaching vital social and conflict-resolution skills.

How to Support Child-Led Turn-Taking

When your child is in the thick of a toy-taking moment, they don't need a lecture or a punishment—they need a coach to help them slow down, take a breath, and navigate the situation. They need you to step in, calmly set limits, and guide them in following through, even when they struggle (and they will in the beginning). Here are four steps you can take to help ease these situations:

1. **Set the Stage:** Explain the expectation in advance, then remind your child in the moment. Instead of saying, "You need to give her a turn," try saying, "You want to play with the doll, and it's not available right now. You can have a turn when he is done."
2. **Offer Support as They Wait:** Don't be afraid of big emotions and tears. This is your child working to accept the limit and processing the disappointment of not having what they want the second they want it. Your toddler is learning impulse control and delayed gratification. Try saying, "I know it's hard to wait." You might also say, "While we wait for our turn, let's see what else we can do!" Waiting isn't easy, especially for toddlers, but offering a distraction or a fun alternative can make the waiting more bearable.
3. **Try a Trade:** The child waiting for their turn can always offer a trade. The child playing can accept or reject it, but it's worth a try.

4. **Practice Patience:** Like any skill, turn-taking needs practice. It's okay if they don't get it right every time—persistence and consistency are key. Your toddler is still learning how to manage their impulses and emotions, and turn-taking is a skill that is developed with practice.

SCRIPTS FOR COMMUNICATION
Sharing

Scenario

Your child takes a toy from their sibling.

What to Avoid

- Labeling Your Child as Not Nice or Bad: "That's not nice!" or "Stop being so bad!"
- Shaming Your Child for Their Lack of Impulse Control: "You're older than him so you should know better."
- Using Control and Domination to Create Compliance: "Give that back right now!" (or grabbing the object from your toddler).
- Using Fear and Threats to Create Compliance: "If you don't give that back, then you are going to time-out" or "If you don't give that back, then no one will want to play with you."

What to Try Instead

- Creating Connection Through Observing and Describing: "You really wanted to play with the car. You took the car from your sister, and now she is crying."
- Creating Connection Through Validation: "It's hard to wait your turn when you really want to play with something."

CULTIVATING SHARING SKILLS

- **Setting Limits to Address Behavior:** "The car is not available right now. It's time to give it back to her."
- **Following Through on Limits:** "It's hard to give back the toy. You really want to play with it, and it's not your turn yet. You can give it back to her, or I can help you."
- **Teaching Skills (Impulse Control):** "When your sister is playing with a toy, it's not available. This means you can play with something else or wait for it to be available when she is done playing with it."
- **Teaching Skills (Problem-Solving):** "Maybe your sister is willing to make a trade. You can try offering her another toy and see if she is willing to accept it."

Supporting your child through toy struggles isn't about swooping in to fix the problem—it's about empowering them with the tools they need to handle it themself. When you slow down, observe, validate their feelings, set clear limits, and guide them toward problem-solving, you're doing so much more than ending a toy battle. You're helping them build confidence, empathy, and self-control—skills that will carry them far beyond the playroom.

TODDLER TIP
Create a Family Toy Philosophy

Having a clear toy philosophy gives kids a sense of security and predictability. It reduces the constant tug-of-war over what's "mine" and what's "yours" and replaces it with understanding, respect, and clear expectations. When everyone understands the rules around sharing and ownership, it's easier to set expectations and manage playtime peacefully.

> Most families find that a mix of communal toys (everyone can play with everything) and personal toys (loveys and other special items that hold personal meaning), which are "off-limits" to others, works best. Communal toys promote connection and cooperation, while special toys honor individuality. To make this work, you must lay the following groundwork:
> - **Define the Rules Together:** Sit down as a family and decide which toys are for sharing and which are personal.
> - **Create Clear Boundaries:** Special toys can stay in a specific space (like a bedroom) during group playtime. Communal toys live in shared spaces. "This truck is really special to you, so let's put it in your room for safekeeping. Everything else is for playing and sharing."
> - **Teach Respect:** Reinforce that it's okay to have personal items, but also important to take turns with communal ones.

FAQs

My child has a really hard time during playdates with other kids touching his favorite toys. What can we do to help him?

When your child has a beloved toy like their favorite truck, doll, or lovey, it can be helpful to put those items away in their room before the playdate begins. Keep the door shut to ensure these prized possessions are safely out of reach. Knowing their special items are secure can help your child relax and enjoy sharing other toys. Keep in mind that it's normal for toddlers to have difficulty allowing others to play with "their" toys. During this time, they need lots of coaching and practice to develop these skills. Use gentle guidance to help them navigate these situations, and remember—it's just a phase and practice makes progress!

My child took a toy and won't give it back. What should I do?

First, stay calm and avoid labeling your child as "selfish" if they just snatched a toy. Use simple, clear language to set expectations. For example, say, "You really like that toy, and your friend is playing with it. Let's give it back and find something else for you to play with." If your child refuses, you may need to help them give it back. Expect tears if this happens and know that it will get better.

Our baby is crawling now and touching my toddler's toys and knocking over towers. My toddler is getting so upset. How do I help them play together?

It's challenging when a baby is curious and eager to explore while an older sibling just wants to be left alone. In these moments, support your toddler by creating a play space that's out of the baby's reach, such as inside a play yard, on a table, or in their toddler-proofed room with the door closed. This gives your toddler a sense of control and personal space.

You can also involve the baby in a way that feels safe for your toddler. For example, say, "She's so excited to play with you because she loves you so much! How about we give her some blocks to play with right here so she doesn't touch your tower?" Be ready to gently redirect the baby back to her toys as needed. This approach respects both children's needs while fostering positive sibling interactions.

My three-year-old is always taking toys from the baby, who recently turned one. They should know better by now, and I'm getting frustrated. How do I make it stop?

Avoid putting the responsibility solely on the older child. Older toddlers still struggle with impulse control, and it's easy to assume that because one child is older and more physically independent, they should "know better." But the reality is that both your one-year-old and your three-year-old are still in the process of developing impulse control. Your baby is entering toddlerhood and doesn't have much control over their impulses either.

Often, the older child's toy-taking behavior started when the baby was younger and didn't care about toys, so the toddler's behavior went unnoticed. But now that the baby is older and is upset by the toy being taken, the toddler is caught in a habit they've been practicing for over a year. The key here is to guide and coach your toddler through the change, rather than expecting them to automatically know how to act. Set clear limits and consistently reinforce them, offering coaching and practice. It will take time for your toddler to adjust.

RAISING A HELPER

There's something magical about the way toddlers eagerly follow you around the house, eyes wide with curiosity, desperate to be part of the action. Toddlers are natural helpers—it's instinctual. "Me do it!" is their battle cry, and while the thought of letting them water the plants or feed the dog might send a shiver down your spine, there's an opportunity here that's bigger than the messes or the extra time it takes.

Sure, it might feel easier to handle the laundry yourself or zip through feeding the pets, but if you want a school-age child who is intrinsically motivated to help around the house, then it's vital to plant the seed early and involve young children when they first show an interest in helping. In the Montessori philosophy, this is called **practical life work**—engaging children in meaningful, real-world tasks that build skills, independence, and a sense of purpose. Letting them pitch in is about more than teaching them to pour kibble into the dog's bowl; it's about fostering their confidence, their sense of belonging, and their intrinsic motivation to be capable, contributing members of the household—and, eventually, the world.

Inviting Toddlers to Help

At this stage in their development, toddlers are trying to make sense of how the world works. They're watching, imitating, and learning from you constantly. And while they may seem like tiny tornadoes of chaos (which, let's face it, they are), their desire to help comes from a deep-rooted developmental need to be autonomous, feel capable, and have a sense of belonging.

Practice inviting your child into an activity by giving them a task they are excited about and capable of that they can do alongside you—even if they don't do it perfectly! Yes, it's going to be messier. Yes, it's going to take longer. But these moments are about so much more than getting the task done. When you pause to let your toddler help, you're creating a sense of ownership in their home and their responsibilities.

> **Benefits of Inviting Toddlers to Help**
> - meets their need to feel capable
> - gives them a role in the family
> - gives them a chance to practice gross and fine motor skills
> - creates connection and quality family time
> - supports the development of concentration and attention span

Shutting down their excitement to help in these early years can have lasting effects. If we constantly say no or brush them off with a "not right now," what we're really telling them is that their contribution doesn't matter—that helping, experimenting, and learning aren't worth the effort. Over time, that excitement to help fades. By the time they're school-age, that spark of curiosity and willingness to take risks has dimmed. They become less inclined to step up, less eager to pitch in, and more reluctant to engage with tasks that don't bring them immediate pleasure or reward. This is often why parents decide to start paying their kids an allowance to do "chores," believing it's the only way they can motivate their child.

This doesn't mean you have to involve your toddler in *everything*. Sometimes you will be too tired or overwhelmed. Other times, your child will be interested in something else. That's okay! Invite them in when it makes sense. By giving them responsibilities—whether that's placing napkins on the dinner table or putting their shoes away—you're teaching them essential life skills.

Household Tasks for Toddlers

Toddlers are capable of so much more than we give them credit for. Sure, they may not fold laundry with military precision or vacuum without missing a few spots, but that's not the point. The point is that they're learning. And the best part? They're having fun while doing it. Focus on effort, not results. Use encouraging language like "You made your bed all by yourself!" rather than correcting or redoing their work.

To make it easier for you, I've broken down the household tasks that toddlers can help with by categories and areas of life and home. Keep in mind that every child is different, and their ability to complete tasks will grow with time and practice. But the more you involve them, the more capable they'll become. Here are tasks your toddler can help with throughout the home:

In the Kitchen
- stirring, measuring, and pouring ingredients (with supervision)
- unloading groceries from the bag and handing them to a parent
- placing napkins and silverware on the table
- scrubbing vegetables with a brush
- helping to unload items from the dishwasher
- wiping down counters with a damp cloth
- sweeping crumbs into a dustpan
- sorting fruits and vegetables into their correct spots
- adding frozen fruit to smoothies
- cutting fruit or veggies with a child-safe knife
- cracking eggs and mixing ingredients

With Pets
- filling water bowls (small pitchers or cups are perfect)
- scooping pet food into bowls

- brushing the dog or cat
- helping to gather toys or put them back in a basket

In the Laundry Room
- sorting laundry by color (a fun, simple matching game!)
- adding clothes to the dryer
- handing you clothes to put in the washing machine
- pressing buttons to start the washer or dryer (with supervision)
- matching socks
- folding simple items like washcloths, small towels, or socks
- putting their folded clothes into drawers or baskets

Tidying Up
- putting toys back in their designated spots (a great way to teach organization and responsibility)
- emptying small trash bags
- wiping down low surfaces (tables, chairs, windowsills)
- squeegeeing windows or shower doors
- watering plants with a small watering can
- picking up trash and putting it in the bin
- helping to vacuum with a lightweight handheld vacuum
- sweeping with a hand broom and dustpan
- putting shoes away
- arranging flowers

With Baby
- fetching diapers, wipes, or a clean onesie
- gently entertaining baby with a rattle or soft toy
- helping to push the stroller (with guidance)
- carrying lightweight items for outings (like a snack bag)

Ready for your toddler to help but not sure how to get started? Here are six tips for getting your toddler involved.

1. **Start Small:** If you're feeding the dog, maybe your toddler's job is to scoop the food into the bowl while you supervise. The key is to find tasks that are just challenging enough to keep them engaged without overwhelming them.
2. **Be Patient and Set Realistic Expectations:** Things won't go perfectly, and that's okay. The goal isn't perfection—it's participation. Celebrate the effort and progress, even if the outcome isn't flawless.
3. **Model the Task First:** Show your toddler how to do the task before expecting them to jump in. Toddlers are visual learners, so seeing you complete the task will help them understand what's expected.
4. **Praise Their Effort, Not Just the Result:** Focus on the process, not the result. "Wow, you worked so hard to sweep the floor!" Then give a high five! This builds their internal motivation and sense of pride.
5. **Make It Fun:** Turn tasks into games or challenges, like "Let's see how many socks we can match!" or "Can you water all the plants before the timer goes off?" This keeps the activity engaging and creates connection.
6. **Give Them Tools:** Give them tools in their size to do the tasks—like a small hand broom or a Swiffer with one section taken out.

> For a printable list of tasks plus a list of my favorite child-size tools and child-safe cleaning products, visit transformingtoddlerhood.com/bookresources.

> ## SCRIPTS FOR COMMUNICATION
> *Raising a Helper*
>
> **Avoid Saying:** "Stop! That's not how you do it! You're making a mess!"
> **Try Saying:** "Thank you for helping feed the dog. Here's how you scoop the food into the bowl."

The Long-Term Benefits of Toddler Helpers

Allowing your toddler to help with household tasks isn't just about getting chores done—it's about raising a child who feels confident, capable, and eager to contribute. These early experiences of being trusted with real tasks help lay the foundation for a teenager who gladly helps around the house and a future adult who is confident in their abilities, responsible in their actions, and eager to step up and help when needed.

And as a bonus, you're also raising a child who sees household chores not as a punishment or a burden but as a natural, enjoyable part of life—a shared responsibility that everyone in the family takes on together.

So next time your toddler tugs at your pant leg and asks to "help," take a deep breath, grab an extra sponge, and let them dive in. After all, those little hands won't stay little forever—but the skills they learn now will last a lifetime.

FAQs

Should I give my child an allowance for doing chores?

First of all, consider dropping the use of the word *chores*. It carries a heavy, negative connotation. Let's be real—no one gets excited about doing chores! That's why I prefer calling them "family tasks" or "household responsibilities."

Young children are naturally driven by an intrinsic desire to help. Offering money in exchange for these tasks can shift their focus from helping because they care about the family to helping only when there's a reward involved. Over time, they may come to expect payment for contributing, undermining the value of being a team player.

If the goal is to raise kids who contribute out of a sense of responsibility and belonging, tying household tasks to an allowance doesn't align with that. Instead, fostering intrinsic motivation by making helping part of the family culture builds long-lasting values centered on cooperation and contribution.

What if my child refuses to help?

Refusing to help can be a sign they're feeling overwhelmed, tired, or unsure how to start. Try breaking tasks into smaller steps, making helping fun (turn it into a game or race), and offering choices: "Would you rather help put away toys or sort laundry?" Offer the opportunity; don't force. Make it playful and keep it positive.

Chapter 45

WELCOMING A NEW BABY

Bringing a new baby into the family is one of life's most beautiful and exciting milestones—and it's also a *major* adjustment, not only for parents but also for their other children. Kids under five often have a tougher time adapting because toddlerhood is a developmental phase that's profoundly egocentric; sharing doesn't come naturally (see chapter 43, "Cultivating Sharing Skills," for a reminder). "Mine" and "me" might be two of your toddler's favorite words, so sharing the person most important to them (you!) with a new sibling can feel monumental, but it's not impossible.

Bringing Home a New Sibling

Fast-forward to the day the baby arrives home. The moment you walk through the door with that newborn, life as your toddler knows it has forever changed. Even if you've prepared them, it can still feel like a shock. Your toddler might respond with excitement, indifference, or resistance to the news of a new sibling. They may act out, regress to babyish behaviors (hello, sudden potty accidents), or become overly clingy. You might notice more tantrums, separation anxiety, parental preference, and limit-testing behavior. Some kids might seem unfazed at first, only to react weeks later when they realize the baby isn't just a temporary visitor but a permanent new roommate.

> ### Common Toddler Reactions to a New Sibling
> - **Jealousy:** Hitting the baby when you feed it.
> - **Frustration:** Saying "Put the baby back in your belly!"
> - **Excitement:** Hugging, kissing, and squeezing the baby (perhaps too hard).
> - **Denial:** Declaring "That is *not* our baby!"
> - **Overwhelm:** Having tantrums out of nowhere.
>
> Remember: Toddlers communicate their feelings, emotions, and needs through their behavior.

The full spectrum of reactions is valid and normal. It's their way of adjusting to the unfamiliar. A new baby can feel like a threat to their bond with you because they now have to share your attention. This can create feelings of insecurity and big behaviors. This doesn't mean your toddler doesn't love the baby or that they're being "bad"—there's an innate bond between siblings that will develop over time. What it means is that your toddler is struggling to cope with a major life change.

When your toddler says, "I want the baby to go back in your belly," they're really asking, "Do you still love me now that the baby is here?" Their words may be blunt, but the deeper question they're wrestling with is one of security and belonging, as they're not yet sure where they fit in this new family dynamic.

Our instinct might be to respond with logic—"The baby can't go back in"—but they really need us to meet them where they are emotionally. Try responding with empathy: "You're wishing things could go back to the way they were before the baby came. It's really hard to share Mommy sometimes, isn't it? I love you no matter what."

The adjustment period varies, but on average, it can take anywhere from a few weeks to a few months. Some toddlers may express their emotions in waves, adjusting at first but then hitting a rough patch later. Others may take longer to warm up to the baby, particularly if the newborn is high needs or if the toddler is naturally more sensitive or slow to warm up in temperament.

With understanding, patience, and intentional support, you can help your toddler navigate this transition, strengthening their emotional resilience and nurturing a loving sibling bond in the process.

Preparing Your Toddler for a New Sibling

The truth is, nothing can fully prepare a toddler for what life will look like once the baby arrives. But you can help pave the way. Begin by introducing the idea in small, digestible ways. Instead of diving into complex conversations about siblinghood, keep it simple and relatable. Talk about the baby in ways they'll understand: "When the baby comes, they're going to need lots of cuddles and naps. We can all cuddle together." This frames the baby as part of a shared family experience, rather than as a stranger who's about to steal all the attention.

Practical Tools

- **Use Stories:** Read books about new siblings to help your toddler visualize what's coming.

> For a list of my favorite books to help your toddler prepare for a new baby, visit transformingtoddlerhood.com/bookresources.

- **Involve Them:** Let them help with baby preparations. Toddlers love feeling useful, and letting them choose a blanket or pick out a baby toy can foster excitement rather than dread.
- **Practice with a Doll:** Role-play with a baby doll. Show your toddler how to gently hold, kiss, and care for the baby. This gives them a sense of control and inclusion.
- **Spend Time with Babies:** Arrange playdates or visits with friends or family who have babies. Seeing real-life interactions

can help your toddler understand what to expect and feel more comfortable.

By involving them in the anticipation and preparation process, you're subtly shifting the narrative from "I'm losing my place" to "I'm gaining a new role."

> ### TODDLER TIP
> *Introduce Baby Dolls*
>
> A great way to help your toddler grasp that a baby is coming home to live with them is to give them their very own baby doll. Here are a few ways baby dolls can be used to help with the transition:
> - Baby dolls give your toddler the opportunity to name their own baby with your full support. "Jelly Space Ranger is a great name!"
> - Your toddler can care for their baby doll when you have an infant to feed, bathe, and put to bed. You can say things like "It's time for Mommy to put baby sister down for her nap. Would you like to put your baby down for their nap too?" This gives them an activity to focus on while you're with baby sister.
> - It provides your toddler ample practice with learning gentle touches and where they can touch their baby sibling when they arrive home.

Helping Your Toddler Adjust to a New Baby

This is the heart of it all. Your toddler isn't just asking, "Do you love me?" They're asking, "Can you love me *and* the baby at the same time?"

The best way to answer that is by making sure they feel seen, heard, and valued in their own right—independent of the baby. Here are seven tools to help:

1. **Verbalize Your Love Out Loud:** Your toddler craves reassurance that your love for them hasn't changed with the arrival of their sibling. You might think your love is obvious, but your toddler needs to *hear* that it's unconditional. Frequent, loving reminders like "I love you so much, and I always will" help to ease their insecurities.
2. **Double Snuggles with Toddler and Baby:** Physical connection is just as powerful as verbal connection, and one of the best ways to help your toddler adjust is through "double snuggles." Create moments where you can cuddle with both your toddler and the baby at the same time. Whether it's reading a story together with the baby nestled in one arm and your toddler in the other, or all snuggled up together on the couch, these moments of closeness will make your toddler feel included rather than pushed aside.
3. **Involve the Baby in Play:** If you're playing with your toddler, have the baby nearby doing tummy time or on your lap. If your baby enjoys being worn, this can free up your hands for playing with or cuddling your toddler. It helps them feel like you're still physically available even when the baby needs attention.
4. **Acknowledge the Behavior You Want to See More Of:** When your toddler is gentle with the baby or plays independently without fussing, acknowledge it. Say things like "I love how kind you were with your baby sister" or "You played so nicely while I was feeding the baby!" This positive reinforcement encourages your toddler to repeat those behaviors because they feel noticed and appreciated.
5. **Involve Your Toddler in Baby Care (Without Overdoing It):** Toddlers love to feel helpful, and involving them in small, baby-related tasks can foster a sense of responsibility and capability. Give them age-appropriate jobs like handing you a diaper, singing to the baby, or putting a pacifier back in place. This not only

makes them feel like they're contributing but also builds their self-esteem. The trick is to keep the tasks light and fun, ensuring your toddler doesn't feel overwhelmed or responsible for the baby's care.

6. **One-on-One Time:** Even if it's only ten minutes a day, carve out special time just for you and your toddler. It doesn't have to be elaborate. A short, focused activity where you put the baby down, silence your phone, and give your toddler your undivided attention can work wonders. Think of this as "filling their cup"—it's a way to reassure them that they still matter, even with a baby in the house.

7. **Use Positive Language:** Use positive language when describing their interactions: "Look, the baby loves when you sing!" or "Your baby brother is so happy when you're around." This helps your toddler see themselves as a valued part of the baby's life rather than in competition with the baby for your love.

TODDLER TIP
Don't Blame the New Baby

Refrain from using the baby as an excuse (blaming the baby) for why you can't do something your toddler wants you to do. Using the baby as an excuse (even if the baby does need you in that moment) can fuel feelings of resentment and frustration toward the new sibling who is consuming a parent's attention, which makes the adjustment harder for everyone.

Let's be real: Adjusting to life with a new baby isn't just hard for your toddler; it's hard for you too. There will be tantrums, regressions, and possibly some jealousy along the way, but remember that this is all part of the process. Be patient with your toddler and, importantly, with yourself.

Focus on the next step, not meeting the end goal this second. Your toddler doesn't need to be the perfect sibling overnight; they just need time and support to get there. Encourage moments of connection between them—whether it's helping your toddler give the baby a soft toy or letting them "teach" the baby something simple. These early interactions will plant the seeds of a strong sibling relationship. Keep in mind that this adjustment can take weeks, even months, and that's okay. Each small step forward is progress.

And don't forget that you're splitting your attention in a way that's new for you too. Be kind to yourself during this time and recognize that you won't be perfect. You may lose your temper or feel guilty for not having enough time for everyone. That's okay. Acknowledge those feelings, but don't dwell in them. You are a good parent who is doing their best!

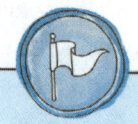

RED FLAG
Postpartum

Having a baby is a big deal. It's vital to look after your physical and emotional well-being first.

During the postpartum period, about 85 percent of women experience some type of mood disturbance. For most, the symptoms are mild and short-lived; however, 10 to 15 percent of women develop more significant symptoms of depression or anxiety.[1]

If you are experiencing symptoms of depression or anxiety or you're just not sure, please contact your doctor or mental health professional and get supported. It's okay to ask for help.

This season of split attention, of jealousy mixed with joy, will eventually smooth out. The love you pour into your toddler, even while you're sleep-deprived and juggling the needs of a newborn, will be felt in their heart. And one day, you'll look over and see them laughing with their sibling—partners in crime, best friends—and you'll know it was all worth it.

FAQs

My toddler is fine until I try to feed the baby. Then they suddenly need everything or start throwing toys everywhere. What can I do?

Talk to your toddler in advance and create a plan for feeding times. Involve older toddlers in making the plan so they feel included. Prepare a special basket of activities that only comes out when you're feeding the baby. Consider having your toddler play on the couch beside you or on the floor nearby. Afterward, discuss how it went during a calm moment and brainstorm ways to make it smoother next time.

My toddler keeps hitting the baby. I keep snapping at my toddler because I want to keep the baby safe, but I think it's making the behavior worse. What should I do?

It's hard not to react when your child's safety is at risk. Instead of saying what not to do ("Don't hit the baby"), show your toddler what you want them to do ("Use gentle hands like this"). Toddlers are still learning how to interact with a new sibling. Hitting may be their way of seeking connection because they don't know how else to engage. It could also be a bid for connection with you. Stay calm and use a discipline approach focused on connection, setting limits on unsafe behavior, and teaching appropriate interaction skills. (See chapter 15, "Redefining Discipline," for more advice on effective discipline.)

My toddler is always so loud when the baby is sleeping—it's almost like she is doing it on purpose. Then the baby wakes up and I'm so frustrated. How do I stop this cycle?

It can feel intentional, but toddlers often struggle with impulse control, especially when they see how much attention the baby gets. Avoid saying, "Shh, you have to be quiet now! The baby is sleeping" or "Don't wake the baby! If you do, you'll be in trouble." Instead, try, "Let's talk in a whisper like this" or "I'm so excited to play—just the two of us. What do you want to do? Maybe we can go outside where it's okay to be loud."

When you tell your toddler no or appear to be attached to a specific outcome, it will trigger your toddler's developmental drive to exert their will and show their independence—inevitably leading to them doing the opposite of what you want. This is what creates power struggles. Try instituting a "quiet time" routine with fun, quiet activities your toddler enjoys while the baby sleeps. Offer positive reinforcement when they remember to be quiet and make it a game where they "help" keep the baby sleeping.

Conclusion

THERE IS NO SUCH THING AS FAILURE

When your child falls while learning to walk, do you view that as a failure? Of course not. You see it as part of the process. Each fall teaches them balance, coordination, and perseverance. The same is true for you. Every time you stumble as a parent, you're gaining the wisdom, patience, and perspective that will guide you forward.

So as we come to a close, let's flip the narrative on one of the biggest lies we tell ourselves in parenting—and in life: the idea that *failure* is something to be feared, something that defines us, something to avoid at all costs. The reality? *There is no such thing as failure.*

Every time you stumble, every time you fall short of your expectations, every time your plans go sideways, you're not failing—you, just like your kiddo, are learning. You're adjusting, adapting, and growing. Mistakes are nothing more than feedback—they are moments that teach you something about yourself, your child, or your circumstances that you didn't know before. If you listen to them, mistakes can become your greatest ally in the messy, beautiful work of parenting.

Redefining "Failure"

Think about those tough moments—the ones that have left you convinced you've messed up beyond repair. Maybe you lost your patience when your toddler threw yet another tantrum. Maybe, instead of the calm, peaceful transition you imagined, bedtime was a disaster filled with tears (yours and theirs). Maybe your parenting-partner dynamic feels like it's unraveling, and every conversation turns into an argument.

In those moments, it's easy to let shame creep in and whisper, *You're not good enough. You've failed.* But what if, instead of seeing these moments as failures, you viewed them as opportunities for growth? What if every time you faced a challenge, you asked yourself, *What is this teaching me?* What if you looked through the windshield of possibility instead of the rearview mirror of regret? Embracing a growth mindset means seeing challenges as opportunities to learn and evolve rather than as fixed limitations or proof of failure. The story you tell yourself in these moments has a big impact on how you view yourself as a parent, how satisfied you are with your parenting journey, and how you respond to your child in challenging moments.

Failure exists only if you let the mistakes stop you. But if you choose to see these moments as steps on the path to becoming a better parent, a better partner, and a better person, failure dissolves into progress. Practice makes progress, not perfection. Remember, you are allowed to learn alongside your toddler.

Here's another secret: There's no such thing as a perfect parent. We all mess up. We all make decisions in the moment that we wish we could take back. But these moments don't define you as a parent—they refine you. They help you see where you need more support, more tools, or just more grace for yourself.

So let's dismantle this myth of perfection. Parenting isn't about getting it "right" every time—it's about showing up, learning, and trying again. Your child doesn't need you to be flawless; they need you to be human. They need to see you navigate challenges, learn from your mistakes, and get back up when you fall. This is how they learn resilience, problem-solving, and the truth that life is a journey of constant growth.

Modeling Resilience for Your Child

When you embrace the idea that there is no such thing as failure, you're not just changing your own perspective—you're modeling something profound for your child. You're teaching them that it's okay to make mistakes, that it's okay to be imperfect, and that growth comes from trying again. This lesson will serve them for the rest of their lives, far beyond their toddler years.

When your child sees you handle tough moments with grace, resilience, and a growth mindset, they learn to do the same. They'll come to understand that mistakes don't define their worth, that challenges are opportunities, and that they have the power to keep going, no matter what.

In the end, we're all toddling along in life. Stay flexible and remember that what feels like a challenge now will probably be a distant memory in a couple of months. Your child is growing and learning at a rapid pace every day, *and* so are you! The journey is not about how many times you fall—it's about how many times you get back up. And every time you do, you're not only becoming stronger but also teaching your child the most important lesson of all: resilience.

So lean into the chaos. Find the love, joy, and meaning woven into the everyday routines, even when they feel relentless. Toddlerhood isn't something to survive—it's something to *experience*. It's an invitation to grow alongside your child, to rediscover patience, and to celebrate every tiny victory—yours and theirs.

As you continue on this parenting journey, remind yourself that you are enough—flaws, stumbles, mistakes, and all. The challenges you face are opportunities for growth, not problems to be solved. There is no such thing as failure; there are only opportunities to learn, grow, and evolve. You are becoming the parent your child needs not by avoiding failure but by embracing it as part of the beautiful, messy process. And I'm here cheering you on!

ACKNOWLEDGMENTS

This book wouldn't exist without a village—the people who believed in me with unwavering support through every messy draft and every moment of doubt.

To my husband—my copilot in life and parenthood—thank you for your patience, encouragement, and countless hours spent holding things down while I poured my heart into these pages. Thank you for holding it all together during all the weekends and late nights when I was writing. You believed in this dream even when I was knee-deep in deadlines and toddler shenanigans, and I'm endlessly grateful for your selfless support.

To my family and friends—thank you for cheering me on, sending "you got this" texts at just the right time, and being a sounding board for ideas when I needed it most. Your support has meant more than I can say (and that's saying something, because I wrote a whole book).

To my agents, publisher, and everyone who had a hand in bringing this book to life—thank you for seeing the heart in this project and guiding it with such care. Your belief turned scribbles and ideas into something real, something I'm so proud of.

To the incredible Transforming Toddlerhood team—thank you for keeping the wheels turning, the emails flowing, and the chaos beautifully managed while I disappeared into writing land. You are the unsung heroes behind every post and project, and I'm endlessly grateful for your talent and dedication.

ACKNOWLEDGMENTS

To the Transforming Toddlerhood community—this is for you. Your stories, your strength, your shared wins and wipeouts, inspired every page. Thank you for showing up, for doing the work, and for letting me walk beside you. I see you covered in crumbs, running on caffeine and very little sleep—this book is yours. May it offer you the comfort of knowing that you're doing better than you think—and you're not alone on this wild ride.

To the tiny humans who make it all so chaotic, so messy, and so deeply worth it—you are the reason we keep showing up, and the reason I wrote this book.

And finally, to my son—my greatest joy and daily reminder of what love looks like in its purest form. Thank you for making me a mother.

Here's to the messy, magical work of raising humans—and growing alongside them.

NOTES

Chapter 2: What Is a Toddler and How Do You Know You Have One?
1. "Toddler Language Development," University of Nevada, Reno Extension, accessed January 30, 2025, https://extension.unr.edu/publication.aspx?PubID=2469.

Chapter 8: Becoming a Safe Parent
1. Elizabeth T. Gershoff, "More Harm than Good: A Summary of Scientific Research on the Intended and Unintended Effects of Corporal Punishment on Children," *Law and Contemporary Problems* 73, no. 2 (2010): 31–56, https://pmc.ncbi.nlm.nih.gov/articles/PMC8386132/.

Chapter 9: Cultivating Patience and Preventing Burnout
1. Amber Thornton, "The Default Parent Syndrome: More Than Just a TikTok Trend," *Psychology Today*, November 14, 2022, https://www.psychologytoday.com/us/blog/the-balanced-working-mama/202211/the-default-parent-syndrome-more-just-tiktok-trend.

Chapter 11: Understanding the Toddler Brain
1. "Brain Development," First Things First, accessed March 19, 2025, https://files.firstthingsfirst.org/for-parents-and-families/brain-development.

2. "Brain Development," First Things First.
3. "Brain Architecture," Center on the Developing Child, Harvard University, accessed April 28, 2025, https://developingchild.harvard.edu/key-concept/brain-architecture/#:~:text=Simple%20neural%20connections%20form%20first,learning%2C%20behavior%2C%20and%20health.
4. "Brain Development," First Things First.
5. "Brain Architecture," Center on the Developing Child.
6. "Brain Architecture," Center on the Developing Child.
7. Daniel J. Siegel and Tina Payne Bryson, "Building the Staircase of the Mind: Integrating the Upstairs and Downstairs Brain," chap. 3 in *The Whole-Brain Child: 12 Revolutionary Strategies to Nurture Your Child's Developing Mind* (Delacorte Press, 2011).
8. Siegel and Bryson, *The Whole-Brain Child*, 38–39.
9. Siegel and Bryson, *The Whole-Brain Child*, 39–40.
10. "Toxic Stress," Center on the Developing Child, Harvard University, accessed March 16, 2025, https://developingchild.harvard.edu/science/key-concepts/toxic-stress/.

Chapter 13: Setting Realistic Expectations

1. "National Parent Survey Overview and Key Insights," ZERO TO THREE, June 6, 2016, https://www.zerotothree.org/resource/national-parent-survey-overview-and-key-insights.
2. "National Parent Survey."

Chapter 15: Redefining Discipline

1. Elizabeth T. Gershoff and Andrew Grogan-Kaylor, "Spanking and Child Outcomes: Old Controversies and New Meta-Analyses," *Journal of Family Psychology* 30, no. 4 (2016): 453–69, https://doi.org/10.1037/fam0000191.
2. *Merriam-Webster Dictionary*, "discipline," accessed March 19, 2025, https://www.merriam-webster.com/dictionary/discipline.
3. Jane Nelsen, "Beware of Logical Consequences," chap. 5 in *Positive Discipline: The Classic Guide to Helping Children Develop*

Self-Discipline, Responsibility, Cooperation, and Problem-Solving Skills (Random House, 2011), 107.

Chapter 18: Teaching Skills

1. Jessica A. R. Logan et al., "When Children Are Not Read to at Home: The Million Word Gap," *Journal of Developmental and Behavioral Pediatrics* 40, no. 5 (2019): 383–86, http://doi.org/10.1097/DBP.0000000000000657.

Chapter 19: Calming an Upset Toddler

1. Shou-Chun Chiang, "Daily Association Between Parent-Adolescent Emotion Contagion: The Role of Parent-Adolescent Connectedness," *Journal of Research on Adolescence* 35, no. 1 (2025): e13038, https://doi.org/10.1111/jora.13038.
2. Britta K. Hölzel et al., "Mindfulness Practice Leads to Increases in Regional Brain Gray Matter Density," *Psychiatry Research* 91, no. 1 (2010): 36–43, https://doi.org/10.1016/j.pscychresns.2010.08.006.

Chapter 20: Transforming Tantrums

1. Andy C. Belden, Nicole R. Thomson, and Joan L. Luby, "Temper Tantrums in Healthy Versus Depressed and Disruptive Preschoolers: Defining Tantrum Behaviors Associated with Clinical Problems," *Journal of Pediatrics* 152, no. 1 (2008): 117–22, https://doi.org/10.1016/j.jpeds.2007.06.030.
2. Sarah M. Coyne et al., "Tantrums, Toddlers, and Technology: Temperament, Media Emotion Regulation, and Problematic Media Use in Early Childhood," *Computers in Human Behavior* 120 (July 2021): 106762, https://doi.org/10.1016/j.chb.2021.106762.

Chapter 23: Responding to Whining

1. Rosemarie Sokol Chang and Nicholas S. Thompson, "The Attention-Getting Capacity of Whines and Child-Directed Speech," *Evolutionary Psychology* 8, no. 2 (2010): 260–74, https://doi.org/10.1177/147470491000800209.

NOTES

Chapter 26: Navigating Screen Time Confidently

1. Chao Li et al., "The Relationships Between Screen Use and Health Indicators Among Infants, Toddlers, and Preschoolers: A Meta-Analysis and Systematic Review," *International Journal of Environmental Research and Public Health* 17, no. 19 (2020): 7324, https://doi.org/10.3390/ijerph17197324.
2. Sudheer Kumar Muppalla et al., "Effects of Excessive Screen Time on Child Development: An Updated Review and Strategies for Management," *Cureus* 15, no. 6 (2023): e40608, https://doi.org/10.7759/cureus.40608.
3. Jenny S. Radesky et al., "Longitudinal Associations Between Use of Mobile Devices for Calming and Emotional Reactivity and Executive Functioning in Children Aged 3 to 5 Years," *JAMA Pediatrics* 177, no. 1 (2023): 62, https://doi.org/10.1001/jamapediatrics.2022.4793.
4. Muppalla et al., "Effects of Excessive Screen Time."
5. Manal M. Alamri et al., "Relationship Between Speech Delay and Smart Media in Children: A Systematic Review," *Cureus* 15, no. 9 (2023): e45396, https://doi.org/10.7759/cureus.45396.
6. Jean M. Twenge and W. Keith Campbell, "Associations Between Screen Time and Lower Psychological Well-Being Among Children and Adolescents: Evidence from a Population-Based Study," *Preventive Medicine Reports* 12 (2018): 271–83, https://doi.org/10.1016/j.pmedr.2018.10.003.
7. Jason G. Goldman, "Sesame Street and Child Development," *Scientific American*, October 15, 2012, https://www.scientificamerican.com/blog/thoughtful-animal/baby-tv-sesame-street-and-child-development/.
8. "Screen Time and Children," American Academy of Child and Adolescent Psychiatry, updated May 2024, https://www.aacap.org/AACAP/Families_and_Youth/Facts_for_Families/FFF-Guide/Children-And-Watching-TV-054.aspx.
9. Brandon T. McDaniel, "Parent Distraction with Phones, Reasons for Use, and Impacts on Parenting and Child Outcomes: A Review of the Emerging Research," *Human Behavior and Emerging*

Technologies 1, no. 2 (2019): 72–80, https://doi.org/10.1002/hbe2.139.
10. Lauren J. Myers et al., "Baby FaceTime: Can Toddlers Learn from Online Video Chat?" *Developmental Science* 20, no. 4 (2016): e12430, https://doi.org/10.1111/desc.12430.
11. Cara D. Goodwin, "Can Young Children Learn from Apps?" *Parenting Translator* (blog), accessed July 9, 2023, https://parentingtranslator.org/blog/can-young-children-learn-from-apps.

Chapter 29: Building Your Child's Confidence
1. Carol S. Dweck, "Inside the Mindsets," chap. 2 in *Mindset: The New Psychology of Success* (Ballantine Books, 2007).
2. Dweck, "Inside the Mindsets," chap. 2 in *Mindset*.
3. Gabriel Araujo, ed., "Your Child's Self-Esteem," Nemours KidsHealth, September 2023, https://kidshealth.org/en/parents/self-esteem.html.

Chapter 30: Cultivating Consent and Body-Safety Skills
1. "The Impact of Sexual Abuse," Praesidium, November 18, 2021, https://www.praesidiuminc.com/why-praesidium/the-impact/.
2. "Child Abuse Statistics," Indiana Center for the Prevention of Youth Abuse & Suicide, accessed January 31, 2025, https://www.indianaprevention.org/child-abuse-statistics.

Chapter 32: Overcoming Sleep Challenges
1. "Child Sleep Duration Health Advisory," American Association of Sleep Medicine, updated April 3, 2016, https://aasm.org/advocacy/position-statements/child-sleep-duration-health-advisory.

Chapter 33: Brushing and Caring for Teeth
1. "Frequently Asked Questions," American Academy of Pediatric Dentistry, accessed July 14, 2025, https://www.aapd.org/resources/parent/faq.
2. "Flossing and Children," Stanford Medicine Children's Health,

accessed July 14, 2025, https://www.stanfordchildrens.org/en/topic/default?id=flossing-and-children-90-P01852.

Chapter 34: Teaching Toilet-Learning Skills

1. Susan Tracy, "Toileting the Montessori Way," Montessori Family Alliance, November 2016, https://www.montessori.org/toileting-the-montessori-way.
2. Kyle A. Richards et al., "Potty Training Before Age 2 Linked to Increased Risk of Later Wetting Problems, Research Shows," Atrium Health, Wake Forest Baptist, October 7, 2014, https://newsroom.wakehealth.edu/news-releases/2014/10/potty-training-before-age-2-linked-to-increased-risk-of-later-wetting-problems-research.
3. Richards et al., "Potty Training Before Age 2."
4. Drew C. Baird et al., "Toilet Training: Common Questions and Answers," *American Family Physician* 100, no. 8 (2019): https://www.aafp.org/pubs/afp/issues/2019/1015/p468.html.
5. Nicole Kavanaugh, interview with Jessica Rolph, "A Montessori Perspective on Potty Learning," Lovevery, accessed July 14, 2025, https://blog.lovevery.com/podcast/a-montessori-perspective-on-potty-learning.
6. "Constipation in Children and Young People: Diagnosis and Management," *NICE Clinical Guidelines*, no. 99 (2017), https://www.ncbi.nlm.nih.gov/books/NBK554924/.
7. Timothy R. Shum et. al, "Sequential Acquisition of Toilet-Training Skills: A Descriptive Study of Gender and Age Differences in Normal Children," *Pediatrics* 109, no. 3 (2002), https://doi.org/10.1542/peds.109.3.e48.

Chapter 35: Ending Mealtime Chaos

1. Gwen Dewar, "The Science of Picky Eaters: Why Do Children Reject Foods?" Parenting Science, November 2022, https://parentingscience.com/picky-eaters/.
2. Caroline M. Taylor and Pauline M. Emmett, "Picky Eating in Children: Causes and Consequences," *Proceedings of the*

Nutrition Society 78, no. 2 (2019): 161–69, https://doi.org/10.1017/s0029665118002586.

3. Grace Fjeldberg, "Raising Healthy Eaters: Should Kids Clean Their Plate?" Mayo Clinic Health System, September 20, 2022, https://www.mayoclinichealthsystem.org/hometown-health/speaking-of-health/raising-healthy-eaters-should-kids-clean-their-plate#:~:text=Introducing%20new%20foods,eat%20more%20than%20one%20bite.

4. Maureen K. Spill, Leann L. Birch, Liane S. Roe, and Barbara J. Rolls, "Eating Vegetables First: The Use of Portion Size to Increase Vegetable Intake in Preschool Children," *American Journal of Clinical Nutrition* 91, no. 5 (2010): 1237–43, https://doi.org/10.3945/ajcn.2009.29139.

5. Trisha Korioth, "Added Sugar in Kids' Diets: How Much Is Too Much?" *AAP News*, March 25, 2019, https://publications.aap.org/aapnews/news/7331/Added-sugar-in-kids-diets-How-much-is-too-much?autologincheck=redirected.

Chapter 36: Balancing Safety and Exploration

1. Ellen Beate Sandseter and Leif Edward Ottesen Kennair, "Children's Risky Play from an Evolutionary Perspective: The Anti-Phobic Effects of Thrilling Experiences," *Evolutionary Psychology* 9, no. 2 (2011): 257–84, https://doi.org/10.1177/147470491100900212.

2. A. D. Pellegrini and Peter K. Smith, "Physical Activity Play: The Nature and Function of a Neglected Aspect of Play," *Child Development* 69, no. 3 (1998): 577, https://doi.org/10.2307/1132187.

3. Rune Storli, "Children's Rough-and-Tumble Play in a Supportive Early Childhood Education and Care Environment," *International Journal of Environmental Research and Public Health* 19, no. 19 (2021): 10469, https://doi.org/10.3390/ijerph181910469, referenced in "Rough and Tumble Play: A Teacher's Guide 2025," *Brightwheel* (blog), January 27, 2025, mybrightwheel.com/blog/rough-and-tumble-play.

Chapter 37: Playing Independently

1. Anna North, "The Decline of American Playtime—and How to Resurrect It," *Vox*, June 20, 2023, https://www.vox.com/23759898/kids-children-parenting-play-anxiety-mental-health.
2. Janelle McArdle, "A Guide to Play Schemas in Early Childhood Education," *Life in a Play Based Classroom* (blog), My Teaching Cupboard, June 5, 2023, https://www.myteachingcupboard.com/blog/a-guide-to-play-schemas-in-early-childhood-education.
3. Richard Larouche et al., "Determinants of Outdoor Time in Children and Youth: A Systematic Review of Longitudinal and Intervention Studies," *International Journal of Environmental Research and Public Health* 20, no. 2 (2023): 1328, https://doi.org/10.3390/ijerph20021328.

Chapter 38: Modeling Manners

1. Craig Smith, "Should You Ask Your Children to Apologize?" *Greater Good Magazine*, Berkeley, September 23, 2016, https://greatergood.berkeley.edu/article/item/should_you_ask_your_children_to_apologize.

Chapter 41: Supporting a Slow-to-Warm-Up (Shy) Child

1. YaeBin Kim and Heidi Petermeier, "Avoid Labeling Your Child," University of Nevada, Reno Extension, 2019, https://extension.unr.edu/publication.aspx?PubID=3011.

Chapter 43: Cultivating Sharing Skills

1. "Teaching Kids to Share," American Academy of Pediatrics, (n.d.), https://www.aap.org/en-us/about-the-aap/aap-press-room/aap-press-room-media-center/Pages/Teaching-Kids-to-Share.aspx, in "Sharing Is Caring . . . AND a Developmental Milestone," *Great Kids* (blog), accessed March 28, 2024, https://www.greatkidsinc.org/sharing-is-caringand-a-developmental-milestone/.
2. Sarah S. MacLaughlin, "Helping Young Children with Sharing," ZERO TO THREE, August 11, 2017, https://www.zerotothree.org/resource/helping-young-children-with-sharing/.

Chapter 45: Welcoming a New Baby

1. Myles Doyle et al., "Perinatal Depression and Psychosis: An Update," BJPsych Advances 21, no. 1 (2015): 5–14, https://doi.org/10.1192/apt.bp.112.010900.

INDEX

aggressive behavior, 250–58
apologizing, 33, 49, 326–29
arbitrary consequences, 110
attachment, 77, 121–22. *See also* connection; separation anxiety
attention deficit hyperactivity disorder (ADHD), 86
attention span, 207, 316–17
autism spectrum disorder (ASD), 86
automatic responses, 50–52

bedtime, 203–4, 259–62, 263–65, 268–69
behaviors
    aggressive, 250–58
    as communication, 4–5, 13, 98–99
    decoder for, 100
    grooming, 242–43
    limit-pushing, 68
    mindset shifts in, 107
    as not good or bad, 95–97
    observing and describing, 96–97
    positive, acknowledging, 112–13
    root of, 98–99
    screen time and, 209
    for sensory needs, 99
    as tip of the iceberg, 97–98
    tracking, during tantrums, 162–63
biting, 12, 252
bodily autonomy, 222, 248, 279
body-safety skills, 241–49
boundaries, 55–56, 189, 222, 227, 243, 245–47, 320, 366
brain, 44–45, 57–58, 73–79, 81, 99, 136, 160, 205–6
breathing, 150, 151–52

calmness, 52, 53–54, 134, 136–37, 147, 148–53, 162, 186, 264, 357

INDEX

cerebral cortex, 76–78
child-led-turn-taking, 362–65
chores, 374–75. *See also* helping
cleaning, 228–29, 284, 300, 318, 321–22, 372
communication
   from aggressive behavior, 253–54
   automatic, 50–52
   behaviors as, 4–5, 13, 98–99
   with the body, 135
   consistency in, 78
   crying and, 169–70, 172–73
   in developmentally smart parenting, 32–33
   during fearful experiences, 148
   hidden messages in, 103–5
   of hurtful words, 191–97
   intentional, 50–52
   interruptions to, 329–30
   negative sentences, 131
   in sibling conflict, 356–57
   skills for, 134–35, 180–81
   threats in, 29–30
   types of, 141, 144
compliance-based approach to parenting, 64
confidence, 231, 235–38, 307, 341
Confident Leader & Guide parent, 35, 37, 41–42
conflict-resolution skills, 132–33, 355, 356–57, 358
connection
   aggressive behavior and, 254, 256
   authentic, 117–18
   at bedtime, 268–69
   brain development and, 74
   choosing over correction, 111
   curiosity in, 120
   in developmentally smart parenting, 34
   in discipline, 105–6
   disrupting the cycle with, 125
   empathy in, 120–21
   making time for, 121
   with new baby and toddler, 380
   overview of, 115
   in parental preference, 203
   physical, 118–19
   playfulness in, 121
   power of, 271
   power struggles and, 219–20
   praise in, 232
   prioritizing, 4
   as relational, 118
   in setting limits, 126
   for sharing, 364
   in sibling conflict, 354–55
   in tantrum response, 161–62
   in toothbrushing, 271
   for transforming behavior, 115–17
   verbal, 119–22
   during whining, 189
   during yelling, 179
connection-based approach to parenting, 64
consent, 241–44, 245–49, 309

INDEX

consequences, 108–11
consistency, 5, 37, 78, 114, 123, 129, 161, 265, 269, 341
constipation, 282, 285
control, 103, 280. *See also* power struggles
Controlling Commander parent, 35, 36, 37, 39, 124
co-regulation, 144–46
crying, 169–73, 174–75

daycare, transitioning to, 342–44
default parent, 56–57
development, toddler, 87–93, 262
developmentally smart parenting, 31–34
discipline, 101–12, 167, 334–35
dressing, 64, 230, 248

early risers, 266, 320–21
eating. *See* mealtimes
emotions
   allowing space for, 229
   avoiding positive dismissiveness in, 143
   brain and, 77
   calmness against, 5
   communication with, 144
   contagion of, 144–45, 155
   contradictory, 167
   co-regulation of, 144–46
   dysregulation of, 141, 154
   empathy for, 5
   FAQs regarding, 153–55
   identifying, 151, 348
   lack of control of, 17
   making peace with, 47
   as not good or bad, 142
   in older toddlerhood, 11
   outbursts of, 153
   reactions to, 50–52
   red flags regarding, 153
   regulation of, 44–45, 130, 133–34
   safety in, 51–52, 53–54, 153–55, 161, 354
   self-care and, 60
   in setting limits, 130
   as signals, 142
   skills, teaching, 133–34, 181
   sleep and, 262
   strategies for, 148–53
   in transitions, 229
   validation of, 33, 120, 134, 142–44, 153–54, 201, 336–37
   in younger toddlerhood, 11
empathy, 5, 120–21, 328
expectations, 88–91, 125, 182, 187, 293–95, 332–33
exploration, 304–9, 310

failure, 236, 385–86
fear, 103, 105, 146–48, 268, 285
fear-based parenting, 30–31, 74–75
fixed mindset, 41, 233
food throwing, 299–300
frustration, 141, 158, 238, 284, 377

403

games, for impulse control, 92
genitals, 244–45, 248–49
greetings, 246, 351
grooming, sexual, 242–43
growth mindset, 41, 233
guilt, 104, 192–93

helping, 369–75, 380–81
highly sensitive person (HSP), 85
hitting, 12, 250, 251, 252, 253, 258, 383
hugging, 241–42
hurtful words, 191–97

"I" statements, 133
impulse control, 91–93, 181, 356, 383–84
independence, 64, 180, 199, 235–37, 272, 311–22
independent play, 147, 311–22, 380
intentional responses, 50–52
interruptions, 329–30

jealousy, 141, 377
judgment, 104–5, 164–65

labels, 95, 178, 232–34, 347
limits, setting
  aggressive behavior and, 254, 256
  big emotions with, 130
  confidence in, 127
  connection in, 126
  consistency in, 114, 123, 129
  in developmentally smart parenting, 34
  in discipline, 106
  follow through of, 126, 129–30
  during hurtful words, 192, 195
  for interruptions, 330
  knowing your role in, 123–25
  leadership in, 126
  at mealtimes, 300
  overcoming challenges with, 129–30
  overview of, 123
  for pacifiers, 274–75
  preserving power of no in, 127–29
  setting clear, 114
  for sharing, 365
  in sibling conflict, 354–55
  for sleep, 266
  success in, 125–27
  in tantrum response, 162
  warnings in, 126
  win-win in, 126
listening, 17, 112
logical consequences, 109–10
love, 18
lying, 334–38

manipulation, 17, 94
manners, 325–33
mealtimes, 214, 246, 293–98, 299–300, 301–3
meltdowns, 81, 89, 116, 157–58, 207. *See also* tantrums

modeling
  of apologizing, 328
  calming tools, 149–50
  in co-parenting, 66
  grounding techniques, 134
  helping, 373
  honesty, 337
  of manners, 325–26
  patience, 330
  of positive language, 195–96, 236
  resilience, 386–87
  for teaching skills, 126, 133
  of toilet usage, 286

Nagging Negotiator parent, 35, 36, 39–40
nail clipping, 220–21
naps, 267, 287–88. *See also* sleep
natural consequences, 108–9, 222
nature, 315–16
new baby, 116, 372, 376–84
night terrors / nightmares, 269
no, 12, 13, 127–29, 223–24

older toddlerhood, 11, 182, 252–53
overwhelm, 57–58, 158, 165, 181–82, 209, 254, 377

pacifier, 274–76
parental preference, 198–204
patience, 55–62, 181, 330, 364
Permissive Pushover parent, 31, 35, 36, 37, 39, 123–24

pets, 299, 371–72
physical safety, 50, 53, 150–51, 161, 354
picky eating, 293, 295–98
play, independent, 147, 311–22, 380
playfulness, 121, 228–29, 273, 305–6, 373
playgrounds, 29, 33, 226, 229–30
pooping, 285–87. *See also* toilet learning
potty training. *See* toilet learning
power struggles, 201, 207, 218–25, 230, 272–74, 295
practical life work, 369
praise, 232–35
preschool, transitioning to, 342–44
problem-solving skills, 135–36

quiet time, 267, 384

reading together, 134–35, 151
redirection, 195, 256–57, 300
reparenting, 46–47
resilience, 231, 237, 386–87
responsive parenting, 77, 78
risky play, 305–7
role-playing, 147, 349
roughhousing, 306, 308–9, 310
routine, 199, 262, 273, 341
routine chart, 236

safe parenting, 48–54
safety, 50, 53, 150–51, 161, 304–9, 310, 353–54

INDEX

scaffolding, 91
screaming, 177–78
screen time, 167, 196, 205–17, 316
secrets, avoiding, 244
self-care, 59–62, 200
self-injury, 164, 166
self-regulation, 145, 160
self-talk, 236
sensory avoiders, 83–84
sensory modulation, 81
sensory overload, 206, 209
sensory play, 317–18, 319
sensory processing, 81, 85–86
sensory processing disorder (SPD), 86
sensory processing sensitivity (SPS), 85
sensory regulation, 82–84
sensory seekers, 82–83
sensory system, 80–81, 82–85, 152, 159, 181–82, 262, 285, 295–96
separation anxiety, 199, 339–45
Sesame Street (TV show), 208
sexual abuse, 242, 245
shame, 103, 104, 284, 307–8, 334–35
sharing, 360–65, 366–68
shyness, 346–52
sibling conflict, 353–59
sign language, 135
sleep, 207, 259–69, 288–90, 383–84
sleep-disordered breathing (SDB), 261, 289
social skills, teaching, 132–33, 181

spanking, 102
strangers, teaching about, 247–48
stress/stress response, 44–45, 77–78, 98–99, 206, 219, 252
swear words, 194–96

tantrums, 5, 12, 88, 94, 156, 157–63, 164–65, 166–68. *See also* meltdowns
teaching skills
  collaboration in, 137
  communication skills in, 134–35, 180–81
  conflict-resolution skills in, 132–33
  in discipline, 106, 107
  emotional regulation skills, 133–34
  emotional skills in, 181
  independence skills in, 180
  overview of, 132
  problem-solving skills in, 135–36
  putting it into practice, 136–37
  social skills in, 132–33, 181
  through modeling, 133
television. *See* screen time
temperament, 99, 346
tickling, 246
time-ins/outs, 111
timer, 227, 320, 331, 361
toddler bed, 267, 272
toddlerhood, overview and characteristics of, 9–13, 14, 15–17, 18–20, 43
toilet learning, 246, 278–92

INDEX

toothbrushing, 270–71, 272–74, 276–77
touching, 243, 245–47, 248–49
toy throwing, 12, 313–14
toys, 315, 316, 319–20, 321–22, 365–66. *See also* independent play
transitions, handling, 226–30, 275, 342–44
tricky people, teaching about, 247–48
trigger(s), 43, 44, 45–46, 158–59, 190

vegetables, 298
video chatting, 215–16, 345
vocabulary, expansion of, 134–35

whining, 94, 184–90
"why" questions, 238

yelling, 75, 176–83
yes space, 315
yes/no questions, 226–27
younger toddlerhood, 11, 182, 185, 252

ABOUT THE AUTHOR

DEVON KUNTZMAN, PCC, is the original toddler parenting coach on Instagram and the founder of Transforming Toddlerhood. As a toddler expert, she is on a mission to transform the myth that toddlerhood is terrible. She has built a community of over one million parents and caregivers from across the world who are committed to transforming their parenting, their toddler's behavior, and their overall experience of toddlerhood while building a relationship with their child that lasts a lifetime.

Through her courses and programs, Devon empowers toddler parents to overcome the challenges of toddlerhood, nurture development, and create confidence in their skills through positive, effective, and developmentally appropriate parenting tools. Since 2018, she has hosted the Transforming Toddlerhood Conference, an esteemed virtual summit for parents featuring renowned parenting experts such as Dr. Shefali Tsabary, Dr. Dan Siegel, and Dr. Tovah Klein. Devon's thought leadership and expertise has been featured in Healthline, Baby List, Motherly, Yahoo! Life, and Fox News.

Devon holds a psychology degree with a focus in child development and is an ICF-certified coach. Additionally, she is a Certified Gentle Sleep Coach and a graduate of the Wonder Weeks Academy Infant Mental Health and Development Program. Having lived on three continents, Devon has tirelessly supported parents and children as a parenting and life coach, former high-profile nanny, and co-director of an orphanage in Rwanda. When she isn't working with parents, Devon can be found playing with her kiddo, riding her bicycle, or drinking a green juice (sometimes all at the same time!).

For additional tips, resources, and tools, visit her website, TransformingToddlerhood.com, or scan the QR code, and follow her on Instagram at @TransformingToddlerhood.